W0050645

Essentials in Ophthalmology

Series Editor

Arun D. Singh

More information about this series at http://www.springer.com/series/5332

Prem S. Subramanian
Editor

Ophthalmology
in Extreme Environments

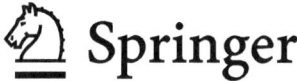 Springer

Editor
Prem S. Subramanian, MD, PhD
Ophthalmology, Neurology, and Neurosurgery
University of Colorado School of Medicine
Aurora, CO, USA

ISSN 1612-3212   ISSN 2196-890X   (electronic)
Essentials in Ophthalmology
ISBN 978-3-319-57599-5   ISBN 978-3-319-57600-8   (eBook)
DOI 10.1007/978-3-319-57600-8

Library of Congress Control Number: 2017943685

© Springer International Publishing AG 2017
This work is subject to copyright. All rights are reserved by the Publisher, whether the whole or part of the material is concerned, specifically the rights of translation, reprinting, reuse of illustrations, recitation, broadcasting, reproduction on microfilms or in any other physical way, and transmission or information storage and retrieval, electronic adaptation, computer software, or by similar or dissimilar methodology now known or hereafter developed.
The use of general descriptive names, registered names, trademarks, service marks, etc. in this publication does not imply, even in the absence of a specific statement, that such names are exempt from the relevant protective laws and regulations and therefore free for general use.
The publisher, the authors and the editors are safe to assume that the advice and information in this book are believed to be true and accurate at the date of publication. Neither the publisher nor the authors or the editors give a warranty, express or implied, with respect to the material contained herein or for any errors or omissions that may have been made. The publisher remains neutral with regard to jurisdictional claims in published maps and institutional affiliations.

Printed on acid-free paper

This Springer imprint is published by Springer Nature
The registered company is Springer International Publishing AG
The registered company address is: Gewerbestrasse 11, 6330 Cham, Switzerland

Preface

This book addresses the challenges faced by humans when functioning outside of the environments considered as "normal" in the modern world. Although our ancestors may have experienced more exposure to heat, cold, sun, water, and wind than does the modern person, there remains a need to be able to function in conditions that fall at the extremes. Certain vocations, such as military service, are more likely to immerse a person in a hostile environment that presents unique barriers to optimal visual function. Heavy industry and construction, among other fields, also routinely pose hazards to the eyes and vision, and injuries to the visual system are both more common than expected for the eye's body surface area and potentially more disabling. Eye protection can mitigate many of these risks, but practical and cultural barriers to the consistent use of these protective devices remain a major challenge.

As if these terrestrial challenges were not enough, humans now can live for extended duration in microgravity, and continued space exploration and life in this completely alien environment may not be possible if a solution to the observed visual changes in microgravity cannot be mitigated. Many terrestrial, aquatic, and avian animals have adapted to life in much harsher environments than are typical for the modern human, and there are many lessons to be learned from the structural and functional differences they exhibit. Finally, even the best-protected eye will sustain injury at times, and we are fortunate to have many techniques available to restore not only anatomical structure but, in many cases, function as well.

Aurora, CO, USA   Prem S. Subramanian, MD, PhD

Contents

Contributors

John Berdahl, MD Vance Thompson Vision, Sioux Falls, SD, USA

Kraig S. Bower, MD Johns Hopkins University, Lutherville, MD, USA

E. Lacey Echalier, MD Department of Ophthalmology, University of Colorado School of Medicine, Aurora, OD, USA

C. Robert Gibson, OD Coastal Eye Associates, Webster, TX, USA

Michael Greenwood, MD Vance Thompson Vision, Sioux Falls, SD, USA

David J. Harris Jr., MD Ophthalmology Division, The University of Tennessee Graduate School of Medicine, Knoxville, TN, USA

Department of Surgery, Knoxville, TN, USA

Thomas H. Mader, MD COL(R), US Army, Cooper Landing, AK, USA

Tana Maurer, BS, ChE, MS EE US Army RDECOM CERDEC NVESD, Fort Belvoir, VA, USA

Michael J. Mines, MD, DVM Madigan Army Medical Center, Department of Surgery, Ophthalmology Service, Tacoma, WA, USA

Christopher O. Ochieng, MD Madigan Army Medical Center, Department of Surgery, Ophthalmology Service, Tacoma, WA, USA

Jeff Rabin, OD, MS, PhD University of the Incarnate Word, Rosenberg School of Optometry, San Antonio, TX, USA

Bruce A. Rivers, MD, LTC Fort Belvoir Community Hospital, Warfighter Refractive Eye Surgery Program and Research Center, Fort Belvoir, VA, USA

Denise S. Ryan, MS Fort Belvoir Community Hospital, Warfighter Refractive Eye Surgery Program and Research Center, Fort Belvoir, VA, USA

Craig Schallhorn, MD LT, MC(FS), USN, San Diego, CA, USA

Steve Schallhorn, MD University of California San Francisco, San Francisco, CA, USA

Carl Zeiss Meditec, Inc., Dublin, CA, USA

Rose Kristine C. Sia, MD Fort Belvoir Community Hospital, Warfighter Refractive Eye Surgery Program and Research Center, Fort Belvoir, VA, USA

Arjuna M. Subramanian Department of Ophthalmology, University of Colorado School of Medicine, Aurora, CO, USA

Prem S. Subramanian, MD, PhD Departments of Ophthalmology, Neurology, and Neurosurgery, University of Colorado School of Medicine, Aurora, CO, USA

Chapter 1
Neuro-ophthalmolmic Sequelae of Sustained Microgravity

E. Lacey Echalier and Prem S. Subramanian

Hemodynamics of Spaceflight

Early in the conduct of space exploration, scientists noted that astronauts developed puffy faces and "bird legs" in the immediate period of spaceflight [37]. The associated stuffy head, headaches, and motion sickness were all grouped into a condition of early spaceflight symptoms called space adaptation syndrome (SAS) or space motion sickness [37]. These conditions are at least in part due to a significant fluid shift which results in central volume expansion and redistribution of fluids from the lower to the upper body during the initial period of weightlessness. In the upright position on Earth (heretofore 1G), veins below the heart hold pressures near 80 mmHg, while venous pressure above the heart is close to zero. In microgravity, the venous pressure will then redistribute throughout the venous system until it theoretically matches the right atrial pressure [4]. There is increased cardiac preload as a result, accompanied by arterial vasodilation and decreased systemic vascular resistance. Interestingly, in one study, the CVP was found to be decreased, while the transmural left ventricular end diastolic dimension was increased [5]. This confirms increased cardiac filling and preload but also demonstrates a paradoxical effect of

E.L. Echalier, MD
Department of Ophthalmology, University of Colorado School of Medicine,
Aurora, CO, USA

P.S. Subramanian, MD, PhD (✉)
Departments of Ophthalmology, Neurology, and Neurosurgery, University of Colorado
School of Medicine, Aurora, CO, USA
e-mail: prem.subramanian@ucdenver.edu

© Springer International Publishing AG 2017
P.S. Subramanian (ed.), *Ophthalmology in Extreme Environments*,
Essentials in Ophthalmology, DOI 10.1007/978-3-319-57600-8_1

microgravity on intravascular pressures. The outcome of these hemodynamic changes is increased stroke volume and overall cardiac output. This phenomenon is further supported by the observations that the heart rate remains relatively unchanged and blood pressure is either the same or slightly lower than preflight measurements. It should also be noted there is a decrease in the plasma fraction after initial central volume expansion stimulates diuresis and the astronauts' bodies subsequently enter a fluid and sodium retaining state [22].

It is not surprising given the cephalad shift and cardiovascular changes that cerebral hemodynamics would similarly be altered. CSF production or drainage in microgravity could theoretically be affected in several ways. Consider that CSF is produced from the choroid plexus and is resorbed in the dural venous sinuses through arachnoid villi, both venous systems. Local venous expansion as seen with cephalad fluid shift could impact CSF balance by means of altering the hydrostatic gradient which determines CSF outflow. Consider the following cerebral hemodynamic relationships: $CBF = (P_a - P_v)/CRV$ where MAP may be substituted for P_a and ICP may be used for P_v. The difference between MAP and ICP represents the cerebral perfusion pressure (CPP). Note that CBF is proportional to CPP and inversely proportional to cerebral vascular resistance (CVR). If the SVR is reduced in spaceflight as discussed above, the associated changes to the CVR would lead to increased CBF. However, fluid shift to the head and neck also could cause poor venous outflow and increase P_v which would cause CBF to decrease. Despite this venous pooling however, the CVP has been shown to *decrease* in microgravity as discussed above; if a similar change occurred in cerebral P_v, then higher CBF might result. The increased cardiac output in microgravity and cephalad fluid shift would increase the P_a and lead to increased perfusion pressure as well if incompletely controlled by autoregulation. The presence of approximately ten times greater pCO_2 aboard the ISS relative to terrestrial atmosphere further complicates these predictions, as elevated CO_2 can lead to chronic vasodilation of cerebral vessels and increased CBF. This is the principle behind the practice of therapeutic hyperventilation in ICU patients to create an acute decrease in ICP.

CBF also is influenced by the unique feature of autoregulation, which in the terrestrial environment would control many of these factors. Head down tilt testing of induced fluid shifts has been attempted to characterize CBF alterations in microgravity. This ground based analog has its limitations, as will be discussed later. Consistent with the above equation, a few studies have given evidence for increased in CBF in HDT. Evaluation of CBF (human) or ICP (rabbit) during HDT showed an immediate rise in CBF or ICP with a slow decline toward pre-HDT baseline, suggesting intact autoregulation in the short term [12, 34]. Conversely, a recent study using phase contrast MRI to measure CBF during short-term HDT on nine healthy subjects found reduced CBF. This was seen even with increased pCO_2 [19]. Data collected on six astronauts pre- and postflight after 1–2 weeks in space also was consistent with acute compensation for microgravity effects through autoregulation [10]. Studies in mice models characterizing histologic features of autoregulation in cerebral vessels demonstrated increased myogenic tone and responsiveness when hind limb suspension was used, but an absence of these autoregulatory changes after spaceflight [9, 35, 36, 38] indicating possible loss of these mechanisms over time in reduced gravity. A complete understanding of cerebral hemodynamics in space-flight continues to be elusive with current testing methods.

Simulation of Cephalad Fluid Shifts

Simulation of weightlessness is a fundamental challenge to researching the physiology of spaceflight. Although weightlessness can be created by parabolic flight providing a very brief period of essential free fall, the period of weightlessness lasts only moments. Research approaches to imitating weightlessness fall into two main categories, head out water immersion (WI) and head down tilt (HDT) bed rest. Water immersion is a logical model in many ways but is impractical for studies aimed at long-duration spaceflight. Head down tilt testing was discovered in the 1970s, when cosmonauts returning home complained they felt they were slipping off the foot of the bed. This problem was alleviated by raising the foot of the bed, and subsequent research identified 6° as the best balance between subject response and comfort [25]. Both methods have their limitations in physiologic effects and practicality. A comparison of the cardiovascular responses during WI or HDT demonstrated similar distention of the atria, increased stroke volume, and suppression of vasoconstrictors, while cardiac output and atrial natriuretic peptide levels were increased more with WI [30]. Furthermore, mean arterial pressure was decreased in HDT and unchanged in WI, similar to decreases in mean arterial pressure seen in long-duration spaceflight [23, 29].

HDT seems to be a natural model for simulation of cephalad fluid shifts in spaceflight; it is not a perfect analog, however, as it creates a shift of gravity vector direction rather than vector neutralization. As previously noted, HDT was used to evaluate CBF in nine healthy subjects and demonstrated an overall decrease in CBF for short-duration studies. Similarly, a murine model using hind limb suspension demonstrated histologic arterial changes consistent with increased autoregulation in cerebral vessels. These findings were absent in mice returned from short-duration (13 days) spaceflight, in which decreased myogenic vasoconstrictor responses and greater vascular distensibility of the basilar and posterior communicating arteries were found [35]. HDT has been used to investigate the ophthalmologic changes seen in spaceflight as well. In a 30-day HDT case study, overall decrease of IOP was reported as well as increased peripapillary retinal nerve fiber layer (RNFL) thickness [33]. Further study of subjects at 14 and 70 days of HDT bed rest demonstrated an increase in the peripapillary retinal nerve thickness in both groups with additional increase shown in the 70-day subjects [32]. However, clinically visible optic nerve edema was not observed in either study. These findings highlight some of the limitations of using HDT as a surrogate testing mechanism for the microgravity environment.

Ophthalmologic Changes Due to Spaceflight

In 2011, the US National Aeronautics and Space Administration (NASA) released a retrospective observational report of ophthalmic findings in seven astronauts who had spent 6 months at the international space station (ISS) [18]. These data were analyzed along with postflight questionnaires of 300 astronauts regarding in-flight vision changes. Six of the seven examined astronauts had nerve fiber layer thickening by OCT and decreased near vision, while five of the seven astronauts had clinically evident optic disk edema and choroidal folds (Fig. 1.1). Five astronauts with decreased near vision exhibited globe flattening on MRI corroborating this change (Fig. 1.2). The refractive changes were not unique to this group. In the postflight surveys, 29% of astronauts on short flight missions complained of degradation of vision while in flight, and 60% of astronauts on long-duration flights complained of the same. Interestingly, three of the seven examined astronauts also exhibited cotton wool spots.

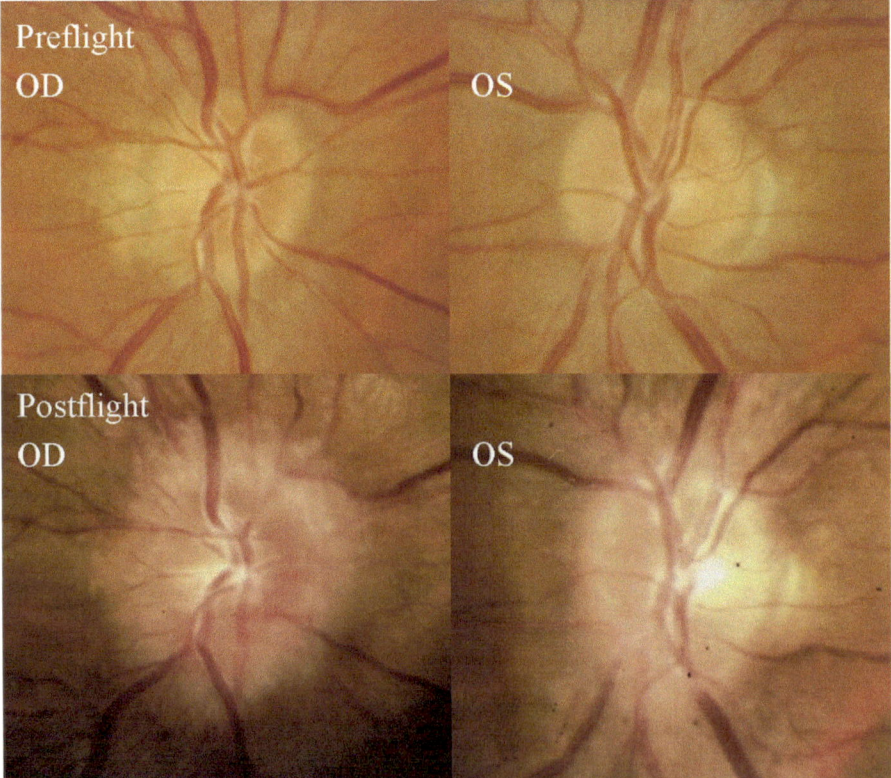

Fig. 1.1 Preflight and postflight optic nerve photos exhibiting optic nerve head edema in an astronaut following long-duration spaceflight (Reprinted with permission from Mader et al. [18])

Fig. 1.2 Postflight choroidal folds (indicated by *arrows*) in both eyes of an astronaut following long-duration spaceflight (Reprinted with permission from Mader et al. [18])

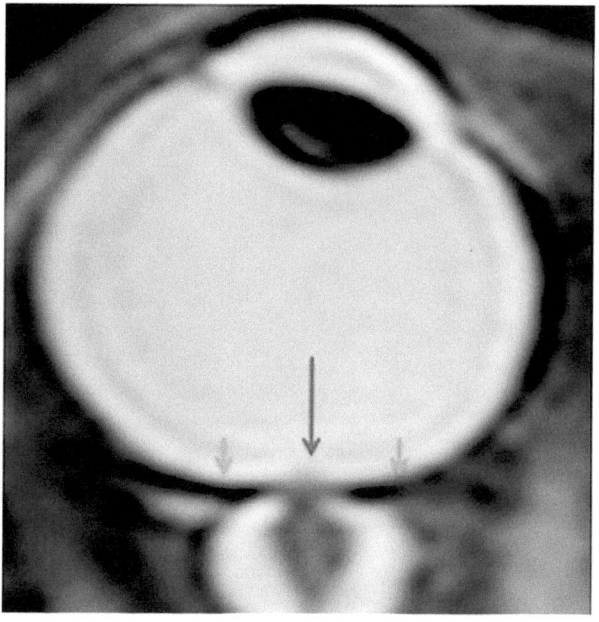

Lumbar puncture was performed in four astronauts of this ISS cohort several days to weeks after their return to Earth. The opening pressures were 22, 21, 28, and 28.5 cm H_2O at 66, 19, 12, and 57 days after mission, respectively. Although these are borderline elevated pressures [1], it is unclear if these ICP readings represent normal variation or the residua of higher ICP while in flight. Beyond this, ICP varies throughout the day much like IOP, so these snapshots may not be representative of the true mean ICP.

The assortment of neuro-ophthalmologic findings associated with spaceflight bears some similarity to the well-characterized condition of idiopathic intracranial hypertension (IIH). Optic disk edema, choroidal folds, increased CSF signal in optic nerve sheaths, and globe flattening with hyperopic refractive shifts are common to both conditions. There are, however, several distinguishing features to suggest that high ICP alone may not be responsible for the observed changes. Astronauts exhibit more impressive choroidal folds and larger hyperopic shifts than those seen in IIH. Further, the imaging used (OCT, MRI, CT, and ultrasound) after long-duration spaceflight demonstrates larger and more persistent shift of CSF into the optic nerve subarachnoid space and more dramatic globe flattening than seen in IIH. Another distinguishing feature is the presence of cotton wool spots, which are not typically associated with IIH. Beyond imaging and examination, the demographics of these two populations are distinctly different, from gender and body habitus to the absence of medications linked to IIH in the astronaut cohort. Finally, the astronauts did not report the associated symptoms that characterize terrestrial IIH, namely, pulsatile tinnitus, diplopia, or chronic severe headaches. In fact, headaches reported by this

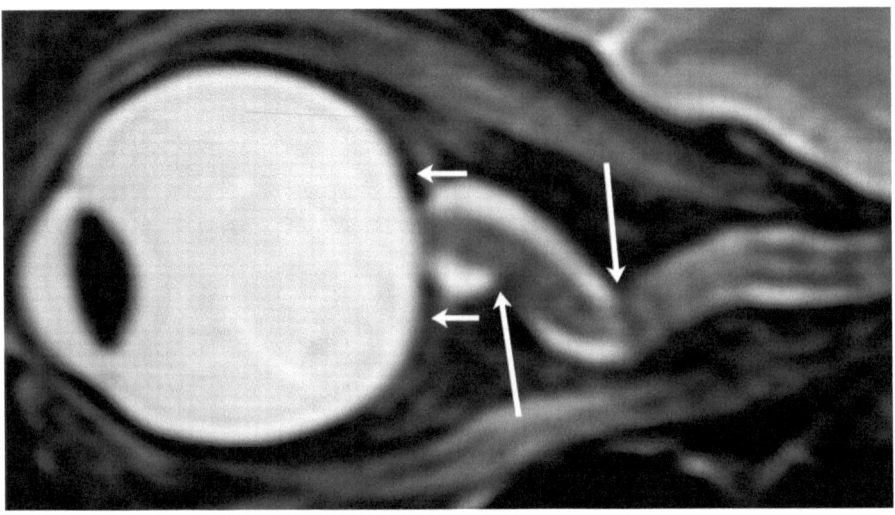

Fig. 1.3 T2 MRI demonstrating optic nerve kinking (*long arrows*) and posterior globe flattening (*short arrows*) (Reprinted with permission, Kramer et al. [14])

long-duration spaceflight group were mild and did not interfere with in-flight activities [18]. This is distinct, however, from the more severe headache experience early in flight as mentioned above.

A follow-up study, in which the postflight MRIs for 27 astronauts after exposure to microgravity were reviewed, found that several exhibited radiologic similarities to those seen in IIH [14]. Posterior globe flattening and optic nerve protrusion were seen in a small subset of these subjects, and moderate concavity of the pituitary dome (partially empty sella) with posterior stalk deviation was also seen in multiple subjects. Increased optic nerve sheath diameter and intrinsic optic nerve enlargement was noted in a small group of subjects. The majority of the subjects demonstrated a central area of T2 hyperintensity within the optic nerve and kinking of the optic nerve sheath as well (Fig. 1.3). A study of MRI images pre- and post-HDT bed rest showed positional and structural changes to the brain, including a shift of the center of mass upward with posterior rotation of the brain and changes in ventricular volume [29]. These changes suggest alterations in CSF homeostasis associated with tissue redistribution.

Given the known relationship between the ophthalmologic findings of disk swelling and retinal nerve fiber layer thickening and increased ICP, as well as the radiologic evidence correlating CNS changes and finally the mild elevation of ICP postflight, NASA has named this syndrome as vision impairment and intracranial pressure (VIIP) [20] .The pathogenesis of optic nerve edema in increased ICP is a mechanical phenomenon in which the pressure along optic nerve sheath becomes elevated. The persistence of optic nerve sheath expansion as well as optic disk swelling for months or years postflight (Mader et al. in press) has led researchers to conclude that CSF dynamics in microgravity may result in permanent changes in optic nerve sheath anatomy. The subarachnoid spaces surrounding the optic nerve are widest at the lamina cribrosa and narrowest in the optic canal. Cisternography with contrast injected directly into the spinal CSF has demonstrated reduced signal beyond the canalicular optic nerve, giving rise to the concept of CSF compartmentalization [13]. This finding challenges the assumption that CSF flow is continuous and equivalent throughout the subarachnoid spaces, cisterns, and ventricles. The relative stasis and trapping of the CSF around the nerve could be further exacerbated by CSF flow changes and positional changes of the brain. Optic disk swelling such as that seen in astronauts may indeed be due to elevated ICP or alternatively by venous engorgement, inflammation, toxicity, metabolic imbalances, or local ischemia. The choroidal folds and hyperopic shift are suggestive of an increase in choroidal thickness as occurs with venous engorgement. This association also provides a possible link between the cephalad fluid shifts and observed ophthalmologic changes.

Vision changes in astronauts create a major safety concern that must be addressed before a planned long-duration spaceflight to Mars (lasting approximately 3 years each way), as these changes could endanger mission success in addition to impacting short- and long-term visual function for individual astronauts. Hyperopic shift is easily correctable by "space anticipation" glasses and has not had a long-term effect on visual potential and function. The crystalline lens is among the most radiosensitive body tissues, and increased terrestrial exposure to ionizing radiation is known to increase the rate of cataract formation. Deep space radiation exposure, which would occur during a flight to Mars, is likely to be even more intense than the exposure received in low-earth orbit (e.g., aboard the ISS), and the potential for accelerated cataract formation exists [7, 8]. While cataract surgery on Earth is one of the most common medical procedures in the developed world, its performance in space or on an alien planet would present formidable challenges. Finally, because we do not understand the etiology of spaceflight-induced optic disk swelling and its persistence in some cases for months after return to the terrestrial environment, the trajectory of this condition (relentless progression vs possible stabilization or even remission as autoregulation occurs) hampers the development of countermeasures that might reduce risk. As a result of the observed changes, NASA is collecting pre-, post-, and inf-light data on the structure and function of ocular and orbital tissues using visual acuity testing, fundus photography, and optical coherence tomography, as well as orbital echography to allow scientists to study changes in a sequential manner and to permit physicians to recognize potentially vision-threatening changes and implement appropriate treatment. To date, no changes have been seen in-flight that would have necessitated medical treatment or other interventions such as early return to 1G, which would have devastating consequences for mission accomplishment.

Study of ICP Changes in Microgravity

Although it is postulated that the visual changes are due to intracranial hypertension, the putative changes in ICP, both short and longer term, have been studied under very limited circumstances. ICP elevation, as noted above, is believed to be occur at least in part because of cephalad fluid shifts. In rabbit studies monitoring ICP by subarachnoid catheter, ICP was immediately elevated from a mean of 4.3 to 8.0 mmHg in 45° HDT reaching a peak of 15.8 mmHg at 11 h but then trended back toward baseline over 7 days [34], suggesting adaptation after the initial spike. Similarly, CBF as measured by transcranial Doppler in humans demonstrated a sudden rise with HDT that decreased toward baseline after 3–6 h in the HDT position [12]. A study of healthy human subjects demonstrated increased ICP after 10 min of HDT as estimated by tympanic membrane displacement [21]; however, similar ICP data are not available from long-duration spaceflight missions. The rapid compensation for the initial ICP rise with HDT implies that autoregulation occurs in the terrestrial environment during HDT; because similar autoregulation may not occur in microgravity as noted above, HDT may not be an adequate model for studying the phenomenon. Furthermore, rodents and rabbits have optic nerve anatomy differences from humans, such as the absence of a lamina cribrosa, that may cause their eyes to respond differently to any changes in CBF and/or ICP.

Because of the concern that ICP might be elevated in space, NASA's Space and Clinical Operations Division as well as affiliated research programs have prioritized efforts to measure ICP either directly or indirectly. A number of methods, some long-standing and others more novel, are being studied as potential methods to be deployed aboard the ISS. Potential strategies include measurement of tympanic membrane displacement, waveform analysis of transcranial Doppler, analysis of otoacoustic emissions, and flow detection within the ophthalmic artery under orbital compression [2, 27]. Many of these methods provide only qualitative data or lack technologic readiness for application in spaceflight at this time. Furthermore, results of noninvasive ICP tests in flight might not be comparable to post- and preflight opening pressures determined by LP. Sampling bias also hampers data analysis, since ICP, like blood pressure and IOP, varies both short term and diurnally. Nonetheless, NASA is committed to measuring ICP in flight and continues to pursue efforts to allow for accurate and meaningful data to be obtained, while protecting astronaut health in flight and minimizing risk to them that could arise during any procedures.

The gold standard for ICP measurement at 1G remains manometric recording of CSF pressure during lumbar puncture in the lateral decubitus position. Equilibration in the manometer can take several minutes if a small bore (less than 23 ga) needle is selected, and the use of a 20 ga needle is recommended [16]. As noted above, postflight LP has been done, but generally days or weeks after return from microgravity. More timely measurement of opening pressure upon return to 1G would be ideal and might be a better indicator of ICP during the final days of the mission, but performing LP immediately on landing is logistically complicated. Not only are there many competing demands on the astronauts' time, but also all returns from the International Space Station presently occur in Kazakhstan (Mader 2016). A standard LP in space would present numerous procedural challenges and risks. There are anatomic changes such as lengthening of the vertebral column and shifting of the nerve roots against the meningeal walls in weightlessness that could increase the risk of procedure complication or failure. Ultrasound assisted LP could mitigate some of these risks but makes the procedure more difficult, possibly requiring a second proceduralist. The aforementioned venous congestion could increase risk of bleeding. Bacterial growth rates and virulence appear to be higher in spaceflight, and the immune system becomes depressed, raising a theoretical increased risk of the microgravity environment. It is unclear if CSF production is normal in space which could inhibit recovery. There are also practical aspects of the procedure such as anchoring of equipment, the patient, and the proceduralist. Classic manometry would not yield useful information as the manometry column is based on Earth's gravitational pull, so digital closed system devices would need to be employed [2]. Given the lack of suitable noninvasive alternatives however, it has been suggested that astronauts be sent into space with a spinal catheter in place. While valuable information might be obtained in this way, a complication such as infection or CSF leak and resultant intracranial hypotension could have devastating consequences in an environment where immediate treatment would not be available. Physicians and scientists continue to struggle with this difficult problem.

Additional contributors to ICP elevation aside from fluid shifts alone must be considered. The blood-brain barrier (BBB) potentially could be compromised, leading to changes in ICP and CBF. The BBB is mediated by specialized endothelial cells lining the cerebral vasculature which are selectively permeable and allow for passive and active transport from the blood into the CSF. Hydrostatic forces, osmotic forces, increased pCO_2, radiation, illness, and a myriad of other factors may influence permeability [20]. Lakin and colleagues created a mathematical model which simulated the intracranial system and cerebrovascular changes of microgravity and demonstrated a hypothetical breakdown in BBB would cause ICP to increase [15]. There is currently no evidence for or against the idea that changes in the BBB are part of the pathogenic process leading to ophthalmic changes in microgravity.

Intraocular Pressure

Abrupt change in body posture from vertical to horizontal or even inverted may cause an acute rise in intraocular pressure (IOP) [26]. This may be due to choroidal vascular engorgement and increased episcleral venous pressure. However, a gradual *decrease* in IOP during prolonged (7–30 days) HDT has been observed [33]. This IOP reduction may be related to a decline in plasma volume that occurs as well during prolonged HDT [6]. A subsequent study of IOP in subjects measured pre- and post-HDT (14 or 70 days) did not find a difference in IOP outcome between the 14- and 70-day groups [32]. In addition, IOP measurements in flight aboard the ISS

Fig. 1.4 Graphic representation of the relationship of IOP and CSF pressure across the lamina cribrosa. (**a**) Represents a balanced or normal TLPG. (**b**) TLPG favoring high pressure on the intraocular side resulting in posterior displacement or cupping as seen in glaucoma. (**c**) TLPG favoring ICP pressure and anterior displacement resulting in papilledema (Reprinted with permission from Berdahl et al. [4])

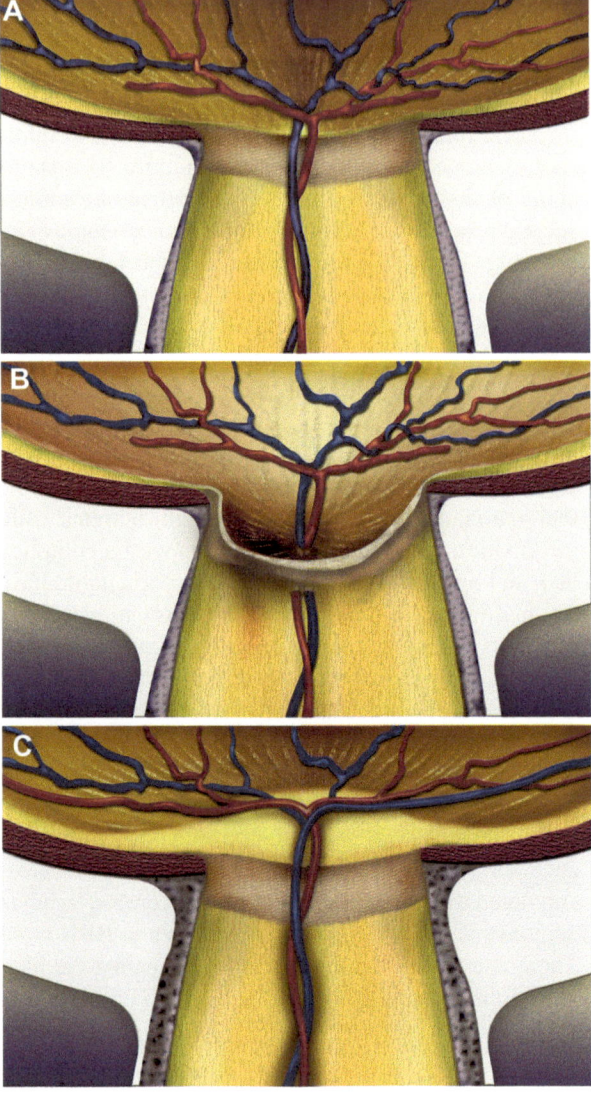

demonstrate a trend toward stable or lower ICP during longer missions without findings of hypotony or visual dysfunction [18]. Homeostasis between ICP and IOP has been proposed to be important for normal optic nerve function and axonal health, as these two opposing forces act on opposite sides of the eye wall at the lamina cribrosa (Fig. 1.4). This translaminar pressure gradient (TLPD) might result in laminar deformation and glaucomatous cupping when IOP-ICP is excessive, while papilledema may occur when ICP-IOP rises. The combination of reduced IOP with stable or potentially elevated ICP in microgravity could increase the TLPD and subject optic nerve axons to injury [4].

The actual role of the TLPD in normal optic nerve function and disease pathogenesis remains controversial. Both retrospective and prospective studies have presented data showing an association between relatively lower ICP and increased risk of developing glaucoma at a given IOP level [3, 28]. A systematic study of the TLPD in subjects with papilledema has not been reported, but a modest correlation between higher severity of papilledema and greater ICP elevation in subjects with IIH has been found [11]. Experimentally induced ICP elevation for 7 days in mice leads to axonal loss and retinal ganglion cell death [24], although the authors could not demonstrate that axonal injury was occurring specifically at the optic nerve head. Ocular hypotony in the terrestrial setting can result in optic disk swelling and choroidal fold formation, two of the ophthalmoscopic findings during long-duration spaceflight. These findings and hypotheses have led researchers to consider seemingly simple countermeasures that could intermittently or even continuously increase IOP to a level that would counter the ICP and restore a "normal" TLPD and thus limit or eliminate the optic nerve changes seen in VIIP.

Conclusions

The VIIP phenomenon presents a formidable obstacle to current aspirations of long-duration space missions or a manned Mars mission. Although there is no conclusive proof of increased intracranial pressure as the causative mechanism, the clinical evidence and similarity of VIIP to terrestrial IIH strongly suggest that ICP elevation contributes to the condition. Increased ICP during spaceflight is plausible in the setting of the known profound cephalad fluid shifts and loss of typical autoregulatory mechanisms in microgravity. Nonetheless, other unknown abnormalities that defy terrestrial physiology may be causative, and careful observation of subjects during long-duration spaceflight remains a crucial task. Unlike in terrestrial IIH, local ischemia or radiation toxicity ultimately may be found to play a role, given the unusual finding of cotton wool spots associated with nerve swelling, choroidal folds, and globe flattening. It has been proposed that the cotton wool spots may represent stresses on the retina similar to high altitude; however, the changes seen at altitude are caused by hypoxia and are more characteristically associated with hemorrhages or Roth spots. We propose that the cotton wool spots may actually represent ischemic injury due to increased radiation exposure in space, a subtle finding in a delicate tissue, which may give us insight into the stresses radiation creates in the astronauts' bodies, but this idea remains a hypothesis without supporting data.

There is a significant research gap due to the lack of terrestrial analogs for study. Human HDT studies and rodent hind limb suspension models have improved our understanding of cephalad fluid shifts of short duration but can neither recreate microgravity nor reveal physiologic changes occurring with prolonged microgravity exposure. This element is key as VIIP was not even observed or known prior to long-duration space missions [31]. The limited number of human subjects available for any studies in microgravity, the competing interests for their time while on the

ISS, and the need to respect their human autonomy and balance individual concerns, needs, and desires against the quest for scientific data cause practical and ethical dilemmas not easily solved. The study of nonhuman primates in microgravity would remove the anatomical limitations (lack of lamina cribrosa, differences in retinal ganglion cell targeting in the brain, etc.) present in studies of rodents and rabbits, but doing so would be exceedingly costly and would raise a new set of practical and ethical concerns.

The use of imaging to characterize optic nerve changes in space has provided important structural data in the absence of ICP monitoring. OCT and serial fundus photos have been collected prospectively since VIIP changes were detected, and NASA is to be commended for expediting the installation of advanced diagnostic equipment aboard the ISS to allow these data to be obtained. OCT of the RNFL is being monitored for changes from preflight values, and postflight OCT tracks the stability or remission of any RNFL swelling (Mader et al. in press). While OCT provides exquisite structural information, it cannot give any functional data. Visual acuity would not be expected to change until very late in the disease process if indeed the optic nerve swelling is similar to terrestrial papilledema, and efforts are in progress to deploy a reliable and sensitive perimetric testing method that would give meaningful functional data that could alert researchers to actual optic nerve dysfunction.

The ultimate goal of this research would be to establish effective countermeasures to vision impairment during and after spaceflight. Interventions determined to be appropriate would preferably be a sustainable single treatment or an effective change in routine as in the rigorous exercise and dietary regimes astronauts undergo. Empiric treatment with acetazolamide has been proposed to ameliorate ICP elevation; however, considering the metabolic derangements, plasma and weight loss in astronauts, this would carry inherent medical risks. It should also be noted that acetazolamide may not even be an effective treatment of VIIP as the pathogenesis is incompletely understood. Additionally, it could lower IOP which would shift the TLPD in favor of disk swelling and choroidal engorgement. A study using lower body negative pressure while in HDT showed attenuation of increases in IOP and ICP [17] which could have positive clinical implications if demonstrated to work in spaceflight. Studies are in progress aboard the ISS to determine if using such devices might be useful in preventing ocular changes. If the pathogenesis of VIIP is confirmed to be increased ICP, more invasive preventative measures could be considered for astronauts being considered for long-duration space missions such as optic nerve fenestration or CSF diversion (i.e., ventriculoperitoneal shunting). Of course, these are very invasive options which would require better understanding of the pathogenesis of VIIP before consideration.

The characterization of VIIP pathophysiology is currently a major priority in space medicine research. The ophthalmologic findings after long-duration spaceflight including optic disk edema, choroidal folds, cotton wool spots, hyperopic shift, and globe flattening with increased CSF signal in the optic nerve sheaths raise significant concern for the preservation of visual function in our astronauts.

It is essential to further characterize the underlying pathology to establish effective and safe countermeasures to resolve this problem in the hopes to create safe passage to ISS, Mars, or beyond.

Compliance with Ethical Requirements E. Lacey Echalier declares no conflict of interest. Prem S. Subramanian has served as a consultant to NASA for the VIIP syndrome. No human or animal studies were carried out by the authors for this chapter.

References

1. Avery RA, Shah SS, Licht DJ, et al. Reference range for cerebrospinal fluid opening pressure in children. N Engl J Med. 2010;363:891–3. doi:10.1056/NEJMc1004957.
2. Barr YR. Lumbar puncture during spaceflight: operational considerations, constraints, concerns, and limitations. Aviat Space Environ Med. 2014;85:1209–13. doi:10.3357/ASEM.3674.2014.
3. Berdahl JP, Allingham RR, Johnson DH. Cerebrospinal fluid pressure is decreased in primary open-angle glaucoma. Ophthalmology. 2008;115:763–8. doi:10.1016/j.ophtha.2008.01.013.
4. Berdahl JP, Yu DY, Morgan WH. The translaminar pressure gradient in sustained zero gravity, idiopathic intracranial hypertension, and glaucoma. Med Hypotheses. 2012;79:719–24. doi:10.1016/j.mehy.2012.08.009.
5. Buckey JC, Gaffney FA, Lane LD, et al. Central venous pressure in space. J Appl Physiol. 1996;81:19–25.
6. Chiquet C, Custaud M-A, Le Traon AP, et al. Changes in intraocular pressure during prolonged (7-day) head-down tilt bedrest. J Glaucoma. 2003;12:204–8.
7. Chylack LT, Feiveson AH, Peterson LE, et al. NASCA report 2: longitudinal study of relationship of exposure to space radiation and risk of lens opacity. Radiat Res. 2012;178:25–32.
8. Cucinotta FA, Manuel FK, Jones J, et al. Space radiation and cataracts in astronauts. Radiat Res. 2001;156:460–6.
9. Geary GG, Krause DN, Purdy RE, Duckles SP. Simulated microgravity increases myogenic tone in rat cerebral arteries. J Appl Physiol. 1998;85:1615–21.
10. Iwasaki K-I, Levine BD, Zhang R, et al. Human cerebral autoregulation before, during and after spaceflight. J Physiol Lond. 2007;579:799–810. doi:10.1113/jphysiol.2006.119636.
11. Kattah JC, Pula JH, Mejico LJ, et al. CSF pressure, papilledema grade, and response to acetazolamide in the idiopathic intracranial hypertension treatment trial. J Neurol. 2015;262:2271–4. doi:10.1007/s00415-015-7838-9.
12. Kawai Y, Murthy G, Watenpaugh DE, et al. Cerebral blood flow velocity in humans exposed to 24 h of head-down tilt. J Appl Physiol. 1993;74:3046–51.
13. Killer HE, Subramanian PS. Compartmentalized cerebrospinal fluid. Int Ophthalmol Clin. 2014;54:95–102. doi:10.1097/IIO.0000000000000010.
14. Kramer LA, Sargsyan AE, Hasan KM, et al. Orbital and intracranial effects of microgravity: findings at 3-T MR imaging. Radiology. 2012;263:819–27. doi:10.1148/radiol.12111986.
15. Lakin WD, Stevens SA, Penar PL. Modeling intracranial pressures in microgravity: the influence of the blood-brain barrier. Aviat Space Environ Med. 2007;78:932–6.
16. Lee SCM, Lueck CJ. Cerebrospinal fluid pressure in adults. J Neuroophthalmol. 2014;34:278–83. doi:10.1097/WNO.0000000000000155.
17. Macias BR, Liu JHK, Grande-Gutierrez N, Hargens AR. Intraocular and intracranial pressures during head-down tilt with lower body negative pressure. Aerosp Med Hum Perform. 2015;86:3–7. doi:10.3357/AMHP.4044.2015.

18. Mader TH, Gibson CR, Pass AF, et al. Optic disc edema, globe flattening, choroidal folds, and hyperopic shifts observed in astronauts after long-duration space flight. Ophthalmology. 2011;118:2058–69. doi:10.1016/j.ophtha.2011.06.021.

19. Marshall-Goebel K, Ambarki K, Eklund A, et al. Effects of short-term exposure to head-down tilt on cerebral hemodynamics: a prospective evaluation of a spaceflight analog using phase-contrast MRI. J Appl Physiol. 2016;120:1466–73. doi:10.1152/japplphysiol.00841.2015.

20. Michael AP, Marshall-Bowman K. Spaceflight-induced intracranial hypertension. Aerosp Med Hum Perform. 2015;86:557–62. doi:10.3357/AMHP.4284.2015.

21. Murthy G, Marchbanks RJ, Watenpaugh DE, et al. Increased intracranial pressure in humans during simulated microgravity. Physiologist. 1992;35:S184–5.

22. Norsk P. Cardiovascular and fluid volume control in humans in space. Curr Pharm Biotechnol. 2005;6:325–30.

23. Norsk P, Asmar A, Damgaard M, Christensen NJ. Fluid shifts, vasodilatation and ambulatory blood pressure reduction during long duration spaceflight. J Physiol Lond. 2015;593:573–84.

24. Nusbaum DM, Wu SM, Frankfort BJ. Elevated intracranial pressure causes optic nerve and retinal ganglion cell degeneration in mice. Exp Eye Res. 2015;136:38–44. doi:10.1016/j.exer.2015.04.014.

25. Pavy-Le Traon A, Heer M, Narici MV, et al. From space to earth: advances in human physiology from 20 years of bed rest studies (1986–2006). Eur J Appl Physiol. 2007;101:143–94. doi:10.1007/s00421-007-0474-z.

26. Prata TS, De Moraes CGV, Kanadani FN, et al. Posture-induced intraocular pressure changes: considerations regarding body position in glaucoma patients. Surv Ophthalmol. 2010;55:445–53. doi:10.1016/j.survophthal.2009.12.002.

27. Ragauskas A, Matijosaitis V, Zakelis R, et al. Clinical assessment of noninvasive intracranial pressure absolute value measurement method. Neurology. 2012; doi:10.1212/WNL. 0b013e3182574f50.

28. Ren R, Jonas JB, Tian G, et al. Cerebrospinal fluid pressure in glaucoma a prospective study. Ophthalmology. 2009; doi:10.1016/j.ophtha.2009.06.058.

29. Roberts DR, Zhu X, Tabesh A, et al. Structural brain changes following long-term 6° head-down tilt bed rest as an analog for spaceflight. Am J Neuroradiol. 2015;36:2048–54. doi:10.3174/ajnr.A4406.

30. Shiraishi M, Schou M, Gybel M, et al. Comparison of acute cardiovascular responses to water immersion and head-down tilt in humans. J Appl Physiol. 2002;92:264–8.

31. Taibbi G, Cromwell RL, Kapoor KG, et al. The effect of microgravity on ocular structures and visual function: a review. Surv Ophthalmol. 2013;58:155–63. doi:10.1016/j.survophthal. 2012.04.002.

32. Taibbi G, Cromwell RL, Zanello SB, et al. Ocular outcomes comparison between 14- and 70-day head-down-tilt bed rest. Invest Ophthalmol Vis Sci. 2016;57:495–501. doi:10.1167/ iovs.15-18530.

33. Taibbi G, Kaplowitz K, Cromwell RL, et al. Effects of 30-day head-down bed rest on ocular structures and visual function in a healthy subject. Aviat Space Environ Med. 2013;84:148–54.

34. Tatebayashi K, Asai Y, Maeda T, et al. Effects of head-down tilt on the intracranial pressure in conscious rabbits. Brain Res. 2003;977:55–61.

35. Taylor CR, Hanna M, Behnke BJ, et al. Spaceflight-induced alterations in cerebral artery vasoconstrictor, mechanical, and structural properties: implications for elevated cerebral perfusion and intracranial pressure. FASEB J. 2013;27:2282–92. doi:10.1096/fj.12-222687.

36. Wilkerson MK, Muller-Delp J, Colleran PN, Delp MD. Effects of hindlimb unloading on rat cerebral, splenic, and mesenteric resistance artery morphology. J Appl Physiol. 1999;87: 2115–21.

37. Williams D, Kuipers A, Mukai C, Thirsk R. Acclimation during space flight: effects on human physiology. CMAJ. 2009;180:1317–23. doi:10.1503/cmaj.090628.

38. Zhang R, Zuckerman JH, Pawelczyk JA, Levine BD. Effects of head-down-tilt bed rest on cerebral hemodynamics during orthostatic stress. J Appl Physiol. 1997;83:2139–45.

Chapter 2
The Effects of Extreme Altitude on the Eye and Vision

Thomas H. Mader, David J. Harris Jr., and C. Robert Gibson

In this chapter, we will review the effects of altitude on the human visual system. In the interest of clarity, we will organize our review based on the anatomic region of the eye and its contribution to visual change during altitude exposure. We will describe the ocular anatomic and physiologic changes associated with altitude exposure and focus on the impact of these changes on visual acuity. When possible, in order to present some historical prospective, we will also include a brief history of how and when these altitude-related visual changes became known. We will also cite examples of how individual patients have been impacted by altitude-related visual changes.

The Cornea

In the normal cornea, constant functioning of an oxygen- and energy-dependent pump in the corneal endothelial monolayer is necessary to maintain corneal deturgescence and clarity. The corneal oxygen supply derives from ambient air, while the nutrients are supplied by the aqueous humor. If this pump is deficient, swelling of the corneal stroma occurs first but does not result in significant opacity. With further endothelial dysfunction, the edema spreads anteriorly into the corneal

T.H. Mader, MD (✉)
COL(R), US Army, Cooper Landing, AK, USA
e-mail: tmader84@gmail.com

D.J. Harris Jr., MD
Ophthalmology Division, The University of Tennessee Graduate School of Medicine, Knoxville, TN, USA

Department of Surgery, Knoxville, TN, USA

C.R. Gibson, OD
Coastal Eye Associates, Webster, TX, USA

© Springer International Publishing AG 2017
P.S. Subramanian (ed.), *Ophthalmology in Extreme Environments*,
Essentials in Ophthalmology, DOI 10.1007/978-3-319-57600-8_2

epithelium, causing profound vision loss and even pain. It is well documented that corneal stromal swelling is an expected physiologic response to high-altitude exposure and occurs as a direct result of hypoxia. A 1996 study done on subjects with normal corneas at 4270 m on Pikes Peak in Colorado described a statistically significant increase in peripheral corneal thickness after 72 h of altitude exposure and a reversal to normal 1 week after return to sea level [32]. In 2007, Morris described a significant increase in central corneal thickness (CCT) in subjects exposed to 5200 m in Bolivia [36]. In 2010 Bosch documented an increase in CCT during a high-altitude ascent to 6300 m in Western China [6]. Specifically, in one group of climbers, the mean CCT increased from 534 to 563 μm, and decreased oxygen saturation was found to parallel the increase in CCT. Their findings suggested that, although the exact cause of the corneal swelling during ascent remains controversial, deficient delivery of oxygen to the aqueous humor may have a role in determining corneal oxygen levels [6]. In a normal cornea, such changes in corneal thickness during altitude exposure are not associated with changes in visual acuity [30]. This is because corneal-derived changes in visual acuity result from either changes in the curvature of the anterior and posterior corneal surfaces or from corneal opacification [35]. Altitude-related corneal edema thickens the normal cornea uniformly, perhaps from depressed endothelial function, but does not impact corneal curvature or clarity. Thus, even though large degrees of corneal thickening may take place during altitude exposure, there is no measureable change in visual acuity in a normal cornea. This contrasts with corneas that have preexisting anatomic abnormalities that may predispose them to develop, in addition to stromal edema, epithelial edema which can then cause corneal opacification during altitude exposure. This was well demonstrated in the 1984 report of a 77-year-old male with low endothelial cell counts who suffered unilateral corneal endothelial decompensation, necessitating corneal transplant, following exposure to 3800 m [22].

Surgical manipulation of the cornea may also set the stage for visual changes during high-altitude exposure. Oxygen to the cornea is thought to be largely supplied by ambient air. As noted above, altitude-related hypoxia causes corneal edema and a uniform increase in corneal thickness but no change in vision. However, surgical alteration of the normal corneal architecture may predispose the cornea to changes in curvature during altitude exposure with resultant visual changes [3, 25–33, 53–55]. This mechanical alteration of normal corneal structure may impact the corneal response to altitude following radial keratotomy (RK), photorefractive keratectomy (PRK), and laser-assisted in situ keratomileusis (LASIK) refractive surgery as well as corneal transplantation.

Effects of Keratorefractive Surgery

RK was performed on millions of active myopic patients during the 1980s and 1990s. The target audience for this procedure was outdoor-oriented young people, to include high-altitude trekkers and mountaineers, who wanted to enjoy the outdoors without the need for glasses. The procedure usually consisted of four to eight radial corneal incisions in the peripheral cornea made at 90% depth with a diamond knife, sparing the central 3–4 mm. This procedure caused a steepening of the peripheral cornea and central flattening, thus decreasing myopia and improving distant vision. Although some degree of diurnal visual fluctuation occurred following this procedure [42], the initial sea level postoperative result was generally satisfactory. However, a very gradual hyperopic shift in refraction often occurs over years in patients after RK [42, 52]. While the surgery is rarely performed today, previously treated patients remain active in outdoor activities and are now aging, making them perhaps even more vulnerable to the adverse effects that altitude may have on their surgically altered corneas.

Following the initial success of the procedure, RK corneas were later found to undergo mechanical changes during altitude exposure leading to changes in vision. Such visual changes have been well documented in the medical literature [9, 28–30, 32, 33, 49] and were also publicized in the book *Into Thin Air* [24] and later mentioned in the movie *Everest*. In one of the early cases, a hyperopic shift and corneal flattening were reported in an RK patient at an altitude of 9000 ft in Aspen, Colorado. The authors hypothesized that the direct mechanical effects of hypobaria were responsible for these changes [49]. Later research, performed in the 1990s, strongly suggested that hypoxia-induced corneal changes were a more likely etiology. Specifically, in 1995, four corneas that had undergone RK were compared to four controls after an overnight stay at two different altitudes in Bolivia [28]. The average increase in cycloplegic refraction spherical equivalent from sea level to 3657 m was +1.03 ± 0.16D and from sea level to 5183 m was +1.94 ± 0.26 D. This study suggested that the RK cornea appears to adjust constantly to changing environmental oxygen concentration, producing a new refractive error over a period of 24 h or more [28]. In contrast, an altitude chamber study in which post-RK subjects were exposed to a simulated altitude of 3660 m for 6 h demonstrated no change in refraction or corneal shape [38]. The extended time to produce visual acuity and corneal contour changes strongly suggests a metabolic origin as opposed to a purely mechanical, pressure-related, phenomenon. This theory was supported by data showing the effect of hypoxia on vision at sea level [63]. Forty subjects (20 post-RK and 20 controls) were fitted with airtight goggles such that one eye was exposed to anoxic conditions (humidified nitrogen, 0% oxygen), and the other was exposed to humidified room air. There was a hyperopic shift of +1.24 D and a +1.19 D change in corneal flattening in RK eyes after only 2 h of exposure to pure nitrogen. RK eyes exposed to humidified room air had no changes in refraction or corneal contour as did the normal eyes exposed to either nitrogen or room air. Both RK and non-RK eyes exposed to pure nitrogen had a significant increase in corneal thickness. All corneas in this study remained clear. These studies all support the notion that the RK visual changes documented during altitude exposure result from the effects of decreased oxygen partial pressure on corneal metabolism and not from the direct mechanical effect of decreased atmospheric pressure. Furthermore, a 2013 study noted that although significant corneal stromal edema was documented in 14 healthy subjects after exposure to 4559 m, there was no change in anterior chamber geometry [59]. This information suggests that the anterior segment anatomy is stable during altitude exposure, and the visual anomalies following RK and other refractive procedures occur solely as a result of corneal changes.

RK alters corneal biomechanics in a distinct manner that, in combination with hypoxic stromal swelling, leads to the characteristic hyperopic shift that has been described. The normal corneal stroma is composed of a meshwork of collagen fibrils extending from limbus to limbus. The collagen fibrils are oriented at various angles to one another in the horizontal plane. This orientation of fibrils contributes to maximum corneal strength within the corneal stroma [28]. Radial keratotomy incisions sever more fibrils that run generally perpendicular to the length of the radial incisions and leave most radially oriented fibrils intact [28]. Since stromal collagen does not completely regenerate after RK, a permanent decrease in corneal strength is predicted [42]. The preservation of radially oriented fibrils and permanent weakening of the circumferential oriented fibrils may lead to an increase in circumferential corneal elasticity. Therefore, as the corneal stroma expands with hypoxia, it remains clear [30], but there is a preferential elevation of the peripheral cornea with central cornea flattening and a resultant hyperopic (farsighted) shift in refraction. Altitude-induced corneal edema and concurrent corneal flattening usually occur only after >24 h at altitude and are not associated with acute exposure [28, 32]. Lid closure during sleep may add to the corneal hypoxia and exacerbate the visual changes [28]. Therefore the visual deterioration in an RK subject may become more evident following a night's sleep at altitude. This may lead to a situation where a high-altitude traveler with RK may wake up in the morning having to cope with an unpredictable change in near and far visual acuity [28, 29, 31].

The impact of these RK-related refractive changes on vision at high altitude appears to be partially dependent on the subject's age. A younger individual has greater accommodative reserve than an older subject and may better compensate for the hyperopic change at altitude. For example, a 20-year-old RK subject was documented to have a +3D shift in cycloplegic refraction from sea level to 5300 m with no subjective visual complaints [27]. In contrast, we documented a 46-year-old RK subject with crisp 20/20 uncorrected distant vision at sea level who experienced an overnight hyperopic shift at 5150 m that resulted in 20/50 distant vision [28]. He also suffered marked near vision loss that left him unable to read his watch, assemble a cook stove, or perform other near vision tasks without assistance [28].

Another important variable in predicting visual disability in RK patients with high-altitude exposure is the postoperative refractive error. An RK climber with residual myopia at sea level may actually enjoy an improvement in distant visual acuity with moderate altitude exposure but note decreasing vision with further exposure to higher altitudes. For example, an RK subject in his 40s with mild myopia at sea level noted an improvement in uncorrected distant vision in Fairplay, Colorado (elevation 3000 m) because his hyperopic shift at this altitude effectively negated his myopia [53]. However, this same individual experienced a decrement in distant vision at 6000 m on a climb in South America and required +1.50D glacier glasses to complete his climb (personal communication, Larry White MD).

Neal Biedelman, a 38-year-old climber with a post-RK sea level refraction of −1.00D, safely ascended Mt. Everest without visual difficulty [27]. His lack of difficulty at extreme altitude was likely due to his baseline myopia and his pre-presbyopic accommodative reserve. In contrast, a 47-year-old RK climber with excellent uncorrected vision at sea level also ascended Mt. Everest but experienced poor near vision and some blurring at distance [33]. Finally, at age 50, Beck Weathers had excellent visual acuity at sea level but experienced a profound loss of vision while attempting to climb Mt. Everest in 1996. Unfortunately, Dr. Weathers did not have a dilated fundus examination after his climb, so it is possible that retinal pathology may also have impacted his visual change [27].

The unique corneal structural changes associated with PRK, LASIK, and corneal transplantation may set the stage for a narrower spectrum of visual changes during high-altitude exposure as compared to RK. Since the late 1990s, PRK and LASIK have largely replaced RK for the surgical correction of myopia and can correct hyperopia and astigmatism as well. PRK reshapes the anterior corneal surface using an excimer laser and does not affect directly the deeper stroma. The Pikes Peak study of 1996 examined the cycloplegic refraction, keratometry, computed video keratography, and central and peripheral corneal thickness in six subjects (12 eyes) who had undergone PRK, six subjects with RK (11 eyes), and nine myopic controls (17 eyes) during 3 consecutive days at 4300 m [32]. Pachymetry measurements demonstrated a significant peripheral corneal thickening in all three groups with a return to normal at sea level. As expected, the RK subjects experienced a significant, progressive, and reversible hyperopic shift in refraction. Subjects who had PRK and those with myopia had no change in refraction [32]. It was hypothesized that although hypoxia caused corneal edema in the PRK corneas, this corneal expansion was uniform across the area of the PRK, and the shape of the anterior corneal surface remained unchanged. Thus, the visual acuity in PRK patients was stable and even appeared suitable for aviators [25]. It is interesting to note that in 2008 an astronaut with bilateral PRKs completed a 12-day Russian Soyuz mission to the International Space Station. Although changing environmental conditions of launch, microgravity exposure, and reentry created an extremely dynamic ocular environment, he reported no visual anomalies [15]. PRK is no longer considered disqualifying for flight personnel in all three military services as well as NASA.

Several studies have examined the stability of post-LASIK surgery corneas during exposure to hypoxia [3, 10, 11, 55]. In the LASIK procedure, a thin flap is created in the cornea and elevated such that the excimer laser can reshape the underlying corneal stroma. The flap is then replaced. Nelson and colleagues used goggles to create an anoxic environment for post-LASIK and normal control eyes and documented symmetric corneal thickening in both LASIK and control subjects as well as a small myopic shift in LASIK corneas [37]. There was a trend toward corneal steepening by keratometry in LASIK subjects, but this was not statistically significant. Such a small myopic shift in an extreme, anoxic environment suggested that LASIK eyes should be relatively stable at high altitude. Several case reports have described variable responses to altitude exposure. White and Boes described

LASIK climbers with decreased distant vision at altitudes of 5947 m and 6961 m, respectively [3, 55]. In contrast one LASIK climber noted no visual change during a climb to 4850 m [10]. Subsequently, Dimmig and Tabin followed six climbers (12 eyes) during a 2002 ascent of Mt. Everest [11]. All had 20/20 vision or better at sea level and maintained this visual acuity at the 5380 m basecamp. One climber reported mild blurring with ascent above basecamp that improved with descent and two other climbers reported blurred vision at 8180 and 8635 m that also improved with descent. Five of the six climbers reported no visual changes up to 8000 m. Three climbers summited the peak (8848 m) with no visual complaints. In summary, these reports suggest that LASIK appears to be a reasonable alternative to glasses, contact lenses, or RK for high-altitude exposure. LASIK is also no longer disqualifying for flight personnel in all three branches of the military and NASA.

Corneal Transplantation

Until about 10 years ago, most corneal transplantation involved the full-thickness trephination and removal of the central portion of a diseased cornea and its replacement with donor graft tissue. Invariably, eyes with such transplants stabilize with about a 50% reduction in the number of viable endothelial cells. Although changes in graft astigmatism and corresponding visual changes are common in the months following a transplant, the vision gradually stabilizes following removal of sutures. A 2001 case report described a successful corneal transplant patient who had stable post-op vision of 20/30 OD with a refraction of plano +2.75 × 030 with all sutures removed approximately 1-year post-corneal transplant for Fuchs endothelial dystrophy [23]. The subject lived at an altitude of 210 m; however, following a 3.5 month stay at 2800 m, the patient's distant vision gradually declined to 20/200 with her spectacles. Manifest refraction was now −6.25 + 3.50 × 055 and best-corrected vision remained 20/30. Five weeks after she returned to her home altitude, she noted an improvement in uncorrected vision and a partial reversal of her myopic shift with a refraction of −3.25 + 2.25 × 050. The authors hypothesized that the relative hypoxia at 2800 m may have caused localized endothelial cell dysfunction and increased circumferential hydration along the graft-host junction. This may have caused an expansion in the peripheral graft with a concomitant central steepening as demonstrated by the rather prominent myopic shift. This case report serves to further illustrate that several varieties of incisional corneal surgeries may predispose patients to visual changes during high-altitude exposure.

More recently, it has become technically feasible to transplant only the stroma in cases of corneal stromal disease and only the endothelium in cases of isolated endothelial dysfunction, although some eyes still require full-thickness transplantation. In general, any patient who has had endothelial transplantation may be at risk of variable refractive status or even corneal opacification when exposed to hypobaric hypoxia.

The Iris and Ciliary Body

While no study has implicated actual dysfunction of the iris at high altitude, abnormalities of pupil dynamics have been described [61]. Transient reduction in percentage change of pupil size, increase in latency, and reduction in speed of contraction were found in climbers reaching 4770 m. These changes were attributed to cerebral effects of hypoxia, but a direct effect on the iris was not considered.

The Trabecular Meshwork

The trabecular meshwork is the primary regulator of intraocular pressure (IOP), which has been investigated extensively in climbers. No study has found glaucoma or other abnormalities of IOP control at high altitude. However, one study found that subjects with higher baseline IOP were at increased risk to develop high-altitude retinal hemorrhages (HARH) later (see below) [7].

The Ciliary Body

The ciliary muscle controls accommodation of the crystalline lens, while the adjacent ciliary processes produce aqueous humor. No abnormalities of either of these functions have been reported to occur at high altitude. However, as noted above, age-related impairment of accommodation (presbyopia) can become acutely manifest and problematic in the setting of a sudden hyperopic shift in a person who has had RK. A decrease in intraocular pressure might be expected in climbers who take acetazolamide to treat or prevent AMS, but this is unlikely to cause visual symptoms. It could theoretically exacerbate retinal, choroidal, and/or optic disc edema, all of which have been reported at high altitude [4, 13, 17].

The Lens

Acute altitude-induced change in the crystalline lens has not been reported. As noted above, refractive changes seen in climbers appear to arise solely from changes in corneal curvature. Indeed, an ultrasonographic study found no change in anterior segment anatomy at high altitude [59]. Long-term ultraviolet (UV) light exposure has been shown to have a weak association with cataract formation [50], so it is possible that the higher ambient UV light at high altitude may hasten the development of cataracts in climbers who do not use adequate UV protection. For climbers who undergo cataract surgery, there is a theoretical advantage in using an artificial lens which blocks both UV and some blue light in order to reduce phototoxicity to the retina [16].

The Vitreous

High-altitude vitreous hemorrhage was first reported in three eyes among 1925 subjects exposed to altitudes between 3300 and 5450 m [47]. In another study, vitreous hemorrhage was the presenting sign of a central retinal vein occlusion that occurred in a climber presumably while at 5300 m; the diagnosis was not apparent until return to low altitude, when the hemorrhage cleared [7]. This climber suffered severe permanent vision loss, but the temporal association of the occlusion with high-altitude exposure cannot be proven, and causation should not be inferred.

The Choroid

The choroid is the pigmented vascular layer that underlies the retina. Increased choroidal thickness has been documented by optical coherence tomography (OCT) in both eyes of a climber who was symptomatic because of a macular hemorrhage in one eye [17]. IOP was not reported, and there was apparently no follow-up after initial evaluation. In essence, this was an incidental finding. As OCT is increasingly able to measure choroidal thickness, asymptomatic choroidal edema may be found to be commonplace in climbers. Interestingly, the degree of thickening in the reported case, 200 μm above the normal 300 μm, was of great enough magnitude to cause or aggravate a hyperopic refractive shift as seen with RK at altitude.

The Retina and Optic Nerve

High altitude has been shown to induce numerous functional and anatomic changes in the human retina since the first description of retinal hemorrhages after high-altitude flights [45] and of high-altitude retinopathy as a component of AMS [47]. The relatively few concurrent studies of native dwellers at moderately high altitudes, such as Sherpas in Nepal who practice agriculture part of the year at up to 5000 m, have noted the relative absence of these findings (Rennie and Morrissey). After ascent to extreme altitudes such as 7000 m, vascular abnormalities are seen in both native and visiting climbers [8]. The anatomical abnormalities will be reviewed first, followed by functional deficits which may be caused by a combination of anatomic and physiologic alterations. The optic nerve is the continuation of the retinal nerve fiber layer and thus will be considered in this section also.

Retinal Vascular Dilatation and Tortuosity

Retinal vascular dilatation and tortuosity have been seen in up to 100% of climbers ascending to 4000 m or higher ([1, 4, 7, 8, 14, 21, 34, 40, 41, 46, 56, 60]). Because there are no known short-term or long- term sequelae, it is appropriate that these findings be labeled a normal physiologic response to altitude. The exact cause is unknown, but recent work has implicated combination of factors. Specifically, increased retinal blood flow in response to hypoxia is thought to combine with relative central nervous system venous obstruction to cause the dilatation, while the tortuosity arises from the mechanical crowding induced by the dilatation [5, 62]. Because this response is so ubiquitous, its occurrence has no predictive or causative relation to AMS. However, one study evaluating AMS found that climbers with high-altitude cerebral edema and small cerebral venous sinuses cannot tolerate even slight increases in cerebral volume, leading to increased intracranial pressure, headache, and papilledema, with increased retinal venous diameter as well [62]. Another study found no correlation between retinal vascular diameter and high-altitude headache [60].

High-Altitude Retinal Hemorrhages (HARH)

First noted by Frayser in 1970, HARH have been found to be commonplace in climbers attaining altitudes over 4000 m [1, 2, 7, 8, 14, 34, 40, 41, 46, 56, 58]. In general, HARH which do not affect the macula are asymptomatic. Like the vascular dilatation described above, HARH have been labeled a normal physiologic response to altitude because of their high incidence. However, since they have been documented to leave mild but permanent sequelae [34, 46, 56], it is more appropriate to refer to HARH as an expected or common response. Interestingly, even in the above reported cases with permanent vision deficit, acute visual symptoms were not reported. The proposed causes are similar to those mentioned above, with the possible additive effect of hypoxia-induced capillary fragility [18]. While HARH have not been definitively associated with concurrent or imminent AMS, one report has found that cerebral deposition of hemosiderin is a marker for previous high-altitude cerebral edema, perhaps implying that microhemorrhages occur in the brain concurrently with those in the eye during high-altitude stress [44]. One study found that climbers with higher baseline line intraocular pressure at low altitude were more likely to develop HARH [7]. Another study cautioned against using HARH as a predictor for AMS, since they were able to document the delayed appearance of HARH after maximal altitude exposure [2].

Retinal Nerve Fiber Layer Infarction

Cotton wool spots, a sign of retinal nerve fiber layer infarction, have been noted in climbers exposed to high altitude [7]. While focal loss of this important retinal layer could result in loss of peripheral vision, no acute symptoms or permanent vision loss were reported.

Disk Edema and Optic Nerve Sheath Enlargement

Disk edema may occur frequently at high altitude, and when seen with vascular dilatation, it may represent a normal response [4]. However, a more recent study by the same group found that parameters associated with increased blood flow and disk edema correlated well with AMS symptoms [5]. Disk edema seen in the setting of true increased intracranial pressure, which correlates with increased optic nerve sheath diameter (ONSD), represents pathologic papilledema. Differentiating papill-edema from disk swelling due to vascular dilatation can be very difficult by ophthal-moscopy alone. Devices to measure increased intracranial pressure noninvasively are not widely available, and measurement of ONSD requires ultrasound or mag-netic resonance imaging (MRI). In one study, ONSD was found to correlate with AMS symptoms and signs, while in another study, this association was found to be insignificant [12, 20].

Color Vision Abnormalities

While no specific complaints from climbers regarding color discrimination have been reported, color vision has been evaluated extensively with various testing methods under both simulated and actual hypobaric hypoxic environments, with most showing mild red-green discrimination deficits. Two studies, one at simulated altitude [48] and the other at 3000 m [19], brought attention specifically to deficits in the tritan axis. The effect was also noted using the Mollon-Reffin Minimalist test in 14 climbers at actual altitudes of up to 5400 m [51]. Subsequently, evaluation of color vision in two climbers at up to 8000 m with a computer-controlled modified Cambridge Colour Test confirmed the tritan deficit at extreme altitude [57]. Both studies showed progressive tritan discrimination loss with exposure to increasing altitude, with delayed but complete return to normal at low altitude. A differential effect of hypoxia on the less numerous S-cones was proposed as a possible mechanism.

Visual Field Abnormalities

Only one study [13] of the potential effects of hypobaric hypoxia on the visual field has been performed at actual high altitude (4559 m). Only the central 20° were tested, and investigators found only a very slight loss of foveal sensitivity. Automated perimetry in simulated high-altitude environments has produced conflicting results. Subjects tested on a Humphrey Visual Field Analyzer showed no visual field changes at a simulated altitude of 3658 m [64]. Another study, using Topcon SBP-3000 perimetry, found a significant drop in peripheral field sensitivity, with a lesser change in central sensitivity, during acute exposure to a simulated altitude of 7620 m. Of note, the authors of the latter study tested only one eye of each subject; during testing, an oxygen mask was not worn, and they judged that reliable conscious response declines after 3–5 min. Thus, the effect of hypoxia alone could explain their findings. Further study of subjects exposed to actual high altitude for realistic periods of time will be required to give meaningful data regarding any deficiency in the visual fields of climbers.

Electroretinographic Abnormalities

ERG responses were investigated extensively in trekkers to 4559 m [43] and alterations in maximum response in scotopic sensitivity, a-wave and b-wave implicit times, implicit times of photopic negative responses, a-wave slope, and i-wave slope were found. The photopic negative response implicit time decrease was found to correlate with arterial oxygen saturation, while the photopic b-wave implicit time correlated with symptoms of AMS. Recovery after return to low altitude was not studied. In contrast, a multifocal ERG study of three climbers to 5650 m found abnormalities in central macular responses persisting 1 week after return to low altitude, but complete return to normal values by 2 weeks [39]. Interestingly, none of these climbers showed HARH. Any clinical significance of these findings remains unknown.

Summary

While research has uncovered many effects of high altitude on the eye, the most important ones are those that impair acute vision to the point of impacting a climber's safety, pose a risk for permanent vision deficit, or serve as a marker for more serious forms of AMS. In the first group, only refractive change after radial keratotomy has been strongly implicated in significant acute loss of sight while climbing, and its mechanism is well understood. High-altitude retinal hemorrhages, while usually benign, can leave permanent scotomata, and central retinal vein occlusion with severe permanent vison loss has occurred at altitude. Finally, controversy exists over the roles of disk edema, retinal hemorrhages, and increased retinal venous and optic nerve sheath diameter as correlates of serious cerebral components of AMS. As with other manifestations of AMS, any symptomatic visual loss at high altitude is best managed by evacuation to lower altitude. This removes the subject from a potentially dangerous environment and may help to prevent further pathologic damage caused by continued altitude exposure.

Compliance with Ethical Requirements Thomas H. Mader, David J. Harris, and C. Robert Gibson declare that they have no conflict of interest. No human or animal studies were carried out by the authors for this chapter.

References

1. Arora R, Jha K, Sathian B. Retinal changes in various altitude illnesses. Singap Med J. 2011;52:685–8.
2. Barthelmes D, Bosch MM, Merz TM, Petrig BL, Triffer F, Bloch KE, et al. Delayed appearance of high altitude retinal hemorrhages. PLoS One. 2011;6(2):e11532.
3. Boes DA, Omura AK, Hennessy MJ. Effect of high-altitude exposure on myopic laser in situ keratomileusis. J Cataract Refract Surg. 2001;27(12):1937–41.
4. Bosch MM, Barthelmes D, Merz T, Bloch KE, Turk AJ, Hefti U, Sutter FKP, Maggiorini M, Wirth MG, Schoch OD, Laudau K. High incidence of optic disc swelling at very high altitudes. Arch Ophthalmol. 2008;126(5):644–50.
5. Bosch MM, Merz TM, Barthelmes D, et al. New insights into ocular blood flow at very high altitudes. J Appl Physiol. 2009;106:454–60.
6. Bosch MM, Barthelmes D, Merz TM, Knecht PB, Truffer F, Bloch KE, Thiel MA, Petrig BL, Turk AF, Schoch OD, Hefti U, Landau K. New insights into changes in corneal thickness in healthy mountaineers during a very-high-altitude climb to Mount Muztagh Ata. Arch Ophthalmol. 2010;128(2):184–9.
7. Butler FK, Harris DJ, Reynolds RD. Altitude retinopathy on Mount Everest, 1989. Ophthalmology. 1992;99:739–46.
8. Clarke C, Duff J. Mountain sickness, retinal heamorrhages, and acclimatization on Mount Everest in 1975. Br Med J. 1976;2:495–7.
9. Creel D, Crandall A, Swartz M. Hyperopic shift induced by high altitude after radial keratotomy. J Refract Surg. 1997;13:398–400.
10. Davidorf JM. LASIK at 16,000 feet (letter to editor). Ophthalmology. 1997;104:565–6.
11. Dimmig JW, Tabin G. The ascent of Mount Everest following laser in situ keratomileusis. J Refract Surg. 2003;19:48–51.
12. Fagenholz PJ, Gutman JA, Murray AF, Noble VE, Camargo CA Jr, Harris NS. Optic nerve sheath diameter correlates with the presence of severity of acute mountain sickness: evidence for increased intracranial pressure. J Appl Physiol. 2009;106:1207–11.
13. Fischer MB, Willman B, Schatz A, Schommer K, Zhour A, Zrenner E, Bartz-Schmidt KU, Gekeler F. Structural and functional changes of the human macula during acute exposure to high altitude. PLoS One. 2012;7(4):e38155.
14. Frayser R, Houston CS, Bryan AC, Rennie ID, Gray G. Retinal hemorrhage at high altitude. NEJM. 1970;282(21):1183–4.
15. Gibson CR, Mader TH, Schallhorn S, Pseudovs, Lipsky, Raid, Jennings, Fogarty J, Garriott R, Garriott O, Johnston. The visual stability of laser vision correction in an astronaut on a Soyuz mission to the International Space Station (ISS). J Cataract Refract Surg. 2012;38(8):1486–91.
16. Henderson BA, Grimes KJ. Blue-blocking IOLs: a complete review of the literature. Surv Ophthalmol. 2010;55:284–9.

17. Hirukawa-Nakayama K, Hirakat A, Tomita K, Hiroka T, Inoue M. Increased choroidal thickness in patient with high-altitude retinopathy. Indian J Ophthalmol. 2014;62(4):506–7.
18. Hunter DJ, et al. Increased capillary fragility at high altitude. Br Med J. 1986;292:98.
19. Karacucuk S, Oner AO, Goktas S, Siki E, Kose O. Color vision in young subjects acutely exposed to 3000m altitude. Aviat Space Environ Med. 2004;75:364–6.
20. Keyes LE, Paterson R, Boatright D, Browne V, Leadbetter G, Hackett P. Optic nerve sheath diameter and acute mountain sickness. Wilderness Environ Med. 2013;24:105–11.
21. Kobrick J, et al. Effects of extended hypoxia on visual performance and retinal vascular state. J Appl Phys. 1971;31:357–62.
22. Koch DD, Knauer WJ, Emery JM. High altitude corneal endothelial decompensation. Cornea. 1984–1985;3(3):189–91.
23. Koe MT, Goodman RL, Waller SG, Johnson DA. Care report: myopic shift in a stable corneal graft following high altitude exposure. Aviat Space Environ Med. 2001;72(12):1145–7.
24. Krakauer J. Into thin air: a personal account of the Mt. Everest disaster. Villard Books, New York; 1997.
25. Mader TH. Guest editorial – Bilateral photorefractive keratectomy with intentional unilateral undercorrection performed on an aircraft pilot. J Cataract Refract Surg. 1997;23(2):145–7.
26. Mader TH. Myopes at altitude: surgical and non-surgical alternatives. Newsletter International Society for Mountain Medicine, Montreal Canada; 1998.
27. Mader TH, Tabin G. Going to high altitude with pre-existing ocular conditions. High Altitude Med Biol. 2003;4(4):419–30.
28. Mader TH, White LJ. Refractive changes at extreme altitude following radial keratotomy. Am J Ophthalmol. 1995;119(6):733–7.
29. Mader TH, White LJ. High altitude mountain climbing after radial keratotomy. Wilderness Environ Med. 1996;1:77–8.
30. Mader TH, White LJ. Corneal thickness changes in very-high-altitude mountaineers. Arch Ophthalmol. 2010;128(9):1224–5.
31. Mader TH, White LJ. Refractive surgery safety at altitude. High Altitude Med Biol. 2012;13(1): 9–12.
32. Mader TH, Blanton, Schallhorn S, Gilbert B, White LJ, Parmley V, Ng J. Refractive changes during 72 hour exposure to altitude following refractive surgery. Ophthalmology. 1996;103(8):1188–95.
33. Mader TH, White LJ, Johnson, Barth F. The ascent of Mount Everest following radial keratotomy. J Wilderness Environ Med. 2002;13(1):53–4.
34. McFadden DM, Houston CS, Sutton JR, Powles AC, Gray GW, Roberts RS. High-altitude retinopathy. JAMA. 1981;245:581–6.
35. McMann, Parmley V, Brady S, White LJ, Mader TH, et al. Analysis of anterior and posterior corneal curvature changes using Orbscan technology in RK eyes exposed to hypoxia. J Cataract Refract Surg. 2001;28:289–94.
36. Morris DS, Somner JE, Scott KM, McCormick IJ, Aspinall P, Dhillon B. Corneal thickness at high altitude. Cornea. 2007;26(3):308–11.
37. Nelson M, Brady S, Mader TH, White LJ, Parmley V, Winkle RK. Refractive changes caused by hypoxia after laser in situ keratomileusis surgery. Ophthalmology. 2001;108:542–4.
38. Ng J, White LJ, Parmley V, Hubickey, Carter, Mader TH. Effects of simulated altitude on post radial keratotomy corneas. Ophthalmology. 1996;103(3):452–7.
39. Pavlidis M, Stupp T, Georgalas I, Georgiadou E, Moschos M, Thanos S. Multifocal electroretinography changes in the macula at high altitude: a report of three cases. Ophthalmologica. 2005;219:404–12.
40. Rennie D, Morrissey J. Retinal changes in Himalayan climbers. Arch Ophthalmol. 1975;93(6): 395–400.
41. Russo A, Agard E, Blein JP, El Chehab H, Lagenaite C, Ract-Madoux G, Dot C. High altitude retinopathy: report of 3 cases. Fr J Ophthalmol. 2014;37:629–34.
42. Schanzlin DJ, Santos VR, Waring GO 3rd, Lynn M, Bourque L, Cantillo N, Edwards MA, Justin N, Reinig J, Roszka-Duggan V. Diurnal change in refraction, corneal curvature, visual

acuity, and intraocular pressure after radial keratotomy in the PERK study. Ophthalmology. 1986;93(2):167–75.

43. Schatz A, Willman G, Fischer MD, Schommer K, Messias A, Zrenner E, Bartz-Schmidt K, Gekeler F. Electroretinographic assessment of retinal function at high altitude. J Appl Physiol. 2013;115:365–72.

44. Schommer K, Kallenberg K, Lutz K, Bärtsch P, Knauth M. Hemosiderin deposition in the brain as footprint of high-altitude cerebral edema. Neurology. 2013;81:1776–9.

45. Sédan J. Hémorrhagies Rétiniennes Survenues Chez Des Hypertendus Au Cours De Vols En Avion. Ann Ocul. 1938;175:307–15.

46. Shults WT, Swan KC. High altitude retinopathy in mountain climbers. Arch Ophthalmol. 1975;93(6):404–8.

47. Singh I, Khanna PK, Srivastava MC, Lal M, Roy SB, Subramanyam CSV. Acute mountain sickness. NEJM. 1969;280(4):175–84.

48. Smith VC, Ernest JT, Pokomy J. Effect of hypoxia on FM 100-hue test performance. Mod Probl Ophthalmol. 1976;17:248–56.

49. Snyder RP, Klein P, Solomon J. The possible effect of barometric pressure on the corneas of an RK patient: a case report. Int Contact Lens Clin. 1988;15:130–2.

50. Taylor HR, West SK, Rosenthal FS, Muñoz B, Newland HS, Abbey H, Emmett EA. Effect of ultraviolet radiation on cataract formation. N Engl J Med. 1988;319:1429–33.

51. Tekavcic-Pompe M, Tekavcic I. Color vision in the tritan axis is predominantly affected at high altitude. High Altitude Med Biol. 2008;9(1):38–42.

52. Waring GO 3rd, Lynn MJ, McDonnell PJ. Results of the prospective evaluation of radial keratotomy (PERK) study 10 years after surgery. Arch Ophthalmol. 1994;112(10):1298–308.

53. White LJ, Mader TH. Refractive changes with increasing altitude after radial keratotomy. Am J Ophthalmol. 1993;115(6):821–3.

54. White LJ, Mader TH. The effects of hypoxia and high altitude following refractive surgery. Ophthalmic Pract. 1997;15:174–8.

55. White LJ, Mader TH. Refractive changes at high altitude after LASIK. Ophthalmology (letter). 2000;107:2118.

56. Wiedman M. High altitude retinal hemorrhage. Arch Ophthalmol. 1975;93(6):401–3.

57. Willman G, Ivanov IV, Fischer MD, Lahiri S, Pokharel RK, Werner A, Khurana T. Effects on colour discrimination during long term exposure to high altitudes on Mt Everest. Br J Ophthalmol. 2010;94:1393–7.

58. Willmann G, Fischer MD, Schatz A, Schommer K, Gekeler F. Retinal vessel leakage at high altitude. JAMA. 2013a;309:2210–2.

59. Willmann G, Schatz A, Zhour A, Schommer K, Zrenner E, Bartz-Schmidt KU, Gekeler F, Fischer MD. Impact of acute exposure to high altitude on anterior chamber geometry. Invest Ophthalmol Vis Sci. 2013b;54(6):4241–8.

60. Willmann G, Fischer MD, Schommer K, Bärtsch P, Gekeler F, Schatz A. Missing correlation of retinal vessel diameter with high-altitude headache. Ann Clin Transl Neurol. 2014;1:59–63.

61. Wilson MH, Edsell M, Imray C, Wright A. Changes in pupil dynamics at high altitude – an observational study using a handheld pupillometer. High Alt Med Biol. 2008;9(4):319–25.

62. Wilson MH, Davagnanam I, Holland G, et al. Cerebral venous system and anatomical predisposition to high-altitude headache. Ann Neurol. 2013;73:381–9.

63. Winkle RK, Mader TH, Parmley V, Polse WLJ. The etiology of refractive changes at high altitude following radial keratotomy: hypoxia versus hypobaria. Ophthalmology. 1998;105:282–6.

64. Yap MKH, Garner LF, Legg S, Faris J. Effects of exposure to simulated altitudes on visual field, contrast sensitivity, and dazzle recovery. Aviat Space Environ Med. 1996;66:243–6.

Chapter 3
Refractive Surgery in Aviators

Craig Schallhorn and Steve Schallhorn

Introduction

> Sometimes, flying feels too godlike to be attained by man. Sometimes, the world from above seems too beautiful, too wonderful, too distant for human eyes to see ... Charles A. Lindbergh, The Spirit of St. Louis, 1953

The cockpit requires complete situational awareness. Vision provides essential sensory inputs regarding flight envelopes and spatial orientation integral to the safety of flight. Visual performance in this setting is vital and must serve the aircrew without fail. Near-perfect visual acuity must effectively and efficiently allow the aviator to maintain a visual scan inside and outside the aircraft, day and night, under hypoxic and hypobaric conditions and in situations when other sensory inputs fail.

Special thanks
Matthew Caldwell, MD, Lt Col, USAF
C. Robert Gibson, OD
Harriet Lester, MD
Thomas Mader, MD
Matt Rings, MD, CAPT, MC(FS), USN
Colonel Scott Barnes, MD, Col, MC, USA
Corina Van De Pol, OD, PhD
Steven Wright, OD, MS

C. Schallhorn, MD (✉)
LT, MC(FS), USN, San Diego, CA, USA
e-mail: csschallhorn@gmail.com

S. Schallhorn, MD
Professor of Ophthalmology, University of California San Francisco, San Francisco, CA, USA

Chief Medical Officer, Carl Zeiss Meditec, Inc., Dublin, CA, USA
e-mail: scschallhorn@yahoo.com

© Springer International Publishing AG 2017
P.S. Subramanian (ed.), *Ophthalmology in Extreme Environments*,
Essentials in Ophthalmology, DOI 10.1007/978-3-319-57600-8_3

In this chapter, the role of corrective lenses and the history and current state of refractive surgery in aviation communities will be discussed. Spectacles and contact lenses remain the most common form of vision correction utilized, but can be ill suited to the physiologic environment of the cockpit, or incompatible with modern avionics equipment. In this setting, refractive surgery plays a pivotal role. The adaptation of refractive surgical techniques into the realm of aviation has been a significant stride forward with potential to improve the safety and performance of aviators in any role.

Vision Correction

Aeronautical medical boards have strictly defined and carefully regulated standards regarding visual acuity dating back to the beginnings of aviation. In most cases, these standards are structured depending on specific flight duties or role of aircrew members (pilot, navigator, student applicant, etc.). FAA civil aviation distant vision standards for Class III general private pilots is 20/40 in each eye, and air transport pilots (Class I) and commercial pilots (Class II) require BCVA (best corrected visual acuity) to be 20/20 in each eye. There are various uncorrected standards for various classes of military aviation personnel, but all military pilots, aircrew and unmanned aerial system operators require best-corrected vision of 20/20 in each eye. Any degradation of best-corrected vision below 20/20 in an eye would require optometric or ophthalmologic evaluation, and a waiver request to higher authority to possibly continue aviation duties. There are additional standards for color vision testing, depth perception, and visual fields.

In years past, aviators were required to have 20/20 uncorrected vision in each eye, and this was the most common medical reason for rejection of aviation applicants. However, visual acuity standards have been gradually relaxed over time, a change driven by many forces, not the least of which are the need to retain aviators and the ability to draw from a larger applicant pool. Incremental lessening of uncorrected visual acuity requirements and refractive standards has produced at least two effects: an increase in physically qualified aviators and new applicants, along with an increase in the prevalence of ametropia [64].

Given the demand for superb visual acuity, refractive error and the need for correction is quite common among aviators. For younger aviators, such as those in military roles, approximately 40% of aircrew will require some form of vision correction. Most aviators over the age of 45 will require some form of correction to maintain near visual acuity due in part to the age-related effects of presbyopia.

The methods for correction of refractive error in the aviation community have evolved over time. At the core of the issue remain corrective lenses: spectacles and contact lenses. However, in the physiologic environments of flight, spectacles and contact lenses have select shortcomings which can limit their effectiveness or even preclude their use. It is in this setting that refractive surgery emerged and essentially redefined the role of vision correction in current aircrew and new applicants alike.

Spectacles

Spectacles have, and continue to be, the predominant method for visual correction. Despite this, spectacles are prone to becoming dislodged, lost, or damaged and may pose a safety issue in extreme circumstances. In a 2001 study, lost or broken eyeglasses were the most common identifiable cause in civil aviation accidents associated with ophthalmic devices [35]. Visually, spectacles restrict field of view, and wearers may experience lens reflections, fogging, or discomfort. Spectacles may not be compatible with integrated helmet systems, or other headwear, such as face masks, chemical defense gear, and night vision goggles. This is especially apparent with pilots of the AH-64 Apache attack aircraft, who utilize a sophisticated helmet-mounted display unit centered over the right eye. This display unit has historically been essentially incompatible with approved eyewear, and a specialized frame was designed to attempt to reconcile incompatibilities. This solution has been regarded as suboptimal, with concerns for comfort and safety, according to a recent study [5].

Pilots of the F-35 Lightning II utilize the Gen III Helmet Mounted Display System (HMDS), which serves as the primary display system, integrating head-up display (HUD), helmet-mounted display, and night vision (Fig. 3.1). Airspeed, altitude, attitude, heading, targeting information and warnings are projected directly to the visor rather than a traditional HUD. This highly specialized piece of equipment is capable of providing augmented reality projections to the pilot, with virtual capabilities to see through the bottom of the cockpit or directly at a target. Image distortion, reflections, and comfort are just a few of the distracting concerns of use with spectacles. The helmet also provides the pilot with active noise reduction, a feature which may be negated with spectacle wear.

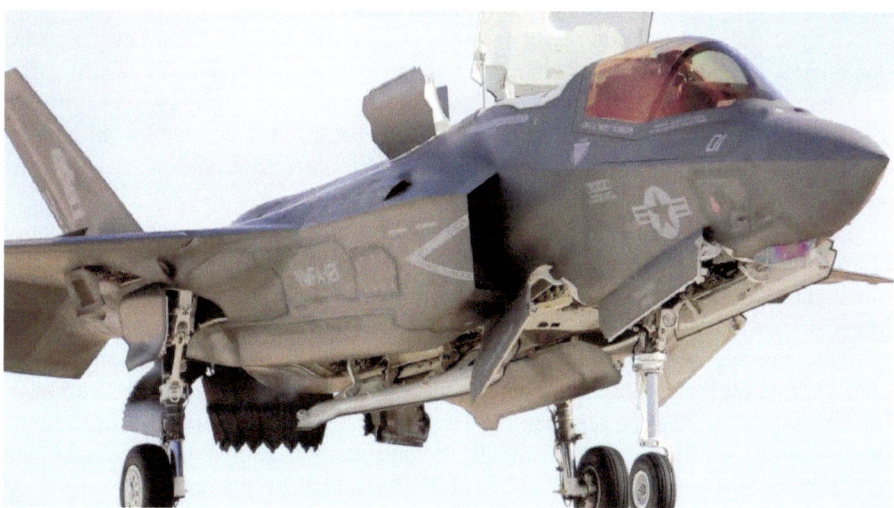

Fig. 3.1 The F-35 Gen III Helmet Mounted Display System integrates head-up display (HUD), helmet-mounted display, and night vision features to provide in-flight and tactical information with virtual capabilities to see through the bottom of the cockpit or directly at a target

Specifically for military aviators, it has long been understood that spectacles would be lost or damaged in an ejection [42]. Additionally, for any pilot downed in theater, the damage or loss of spectacles (or contact lenses) make survival and evasion improbable. Corrective lenses may be taken away by captors to reduce chances of escape. With regard to visual performance, past studies on US Navy jet pilots suggests that aviators who do not require eyewear may be able to identify targets at a greater distance [59], though these aviators tend to perform equally well on an extremely demanding visual task: night carrier landing operations [54].

Contact Lenses

Contact lenses have historically received scrutiny by the aviation community and for good cause. The ocular surface environment experienced by aircrew is hypoxic, hypobaric, very dry with low humidity, with exposure to fumes and circulating particulates, and overall unhygienic conditions that are unfavorable for routine contact lens use [40]. Wear at high altitudes or rapid decompression is known to result in sub-contact lens nitrogen bubbles, which are located at the limbus and not of visual significance for soft lenses, but primarily central for rigid lenses [13]. Low altitude use, particularly in rotary wing aircraft, is associated with high degrees of exposure to particulate matter [63]. For military applications, use in the field or austere conditions makes proper hygiene difficult if not impossible to maintain. Additionally, a study of Navy and Marine ejections from 1980 to 2000 in the Naval Safety Center database showed that the majority of pilots retained their contact lenses during ejection by reflex eye closure, though still suffering some subconjunctival hemorrhages from windblast forces [47].

Despite these shortcomings, a significant body of evidence has been accumulated supporting the safety of contact lenses in aviators [39]. In civil aviation, contact lenses have been approved for use without waiver since 1976. Multifocal contact lenses, used by civil aviators to aid with presbyopia, are subject to medical approval and require 1 month of use before returning to aviation duties to allow for adaptation.

For military aviators, contact lenses were approved following robust evaluation during the 1980s. Soft lenses are available to aircrew by medical support detachments and do not require specific waiver, provided there are no concerning symptoms or complications which may interfere with safety of flight. Aviators need official approval from their local flight surgeon and eye care provider familiar with current contact lens policy and instruction. They are still required to fly with back-up spectacles in case of removal or loss during flight. Aviators who use contact lenses are generally examined annually by an optometrist or ophthalmologist, and any contact lens-related complication is reported and closely monitored. In this context, contact lenses are considered safe and effective refractive options and remain popular among military aviators and their civilian counterparts.

Corneal Refractive Surgery

To a large extent, the adaptation of corneal refractive surgery (CRS) to aviation represented the final frontier for these procedures. Aviators generally have the most stringent visual requirements, and anything which could potentially interfere with flight duties, be it loss of vision or debilitating ocular or visual symptoms as a result of surgery, requires a very cautious approach.

Historically, there have been a number of barriers to the approval of CRS in aircrew. Visual metrics beyond high-contrast Snellen acuity have merited ongoing attention, such as visual performance or low-light acuity, because of the unique operational demands of many aircrew. Low-contrast acuity, night vision, symptoms of glare or halos, corneal haze, or decreased subjective visual performance can have a multitude of unfavorable effects, not the least of which would be concerns about the safety of flight.

Military aircrew of tactical aircraft faces the additional hazard of ejection, which is the most common cause of eye injury in flight mishaps [47]. Post-ejection windblast and flailing equipment or limbs pose serious risks to the eye, and any surgical procedure which could weaken the cornea and possibly predispose the eye to injury must be considered. Furthermore, the operational logistics of a prolonged visual recovery period after surgery can be prohibitive to squadrons and flight operations.

Overall, the use of refractive surgery in aviators is akin to many new medical interventions: the risks of grounding an aviator due to adverse visual outcomes must be weighed against the potential benefits. As such, it comes as no surprise that the early history of refractive surgery did not begin with studies on flight personnel. Rather, prior to US Food and Drug Administration (FDA) approval, as PRK was under study in the United States, the procedure received special scrutiny by the US military for its role in non-aviators, who also face unique and noxious environments despite robust visual needs. The results of these studies, some of which will be discussed, were pivotal in the application of refractive surgery in aviators and flight personnel.

History and Approval of Refractive Surgery in Aviators

Of important historical consideration in the eventual adoption of corneal refractive surgery by the aviation community is radial keratotomy (RK). In RK, a number of deep, radially oriented incisions in the corneal stroma were created using a special diamond knife. The net effect of these incisions was a flattening of the central cornea, reducing the refractive power of the eye for the treatment of myopia. The consequences of this procedure most concerning for aviators were (1) the cornea is less able to withstand even minor trauma, (2) diurnal and long-term refractive instability, and (3) significant refractive changes under hypoxic conditions. A significant, but reversible, hyperopic shift in refractive error has been observed following RK under hypoxic conditions [27]. RK incisions also cause loss of corneal endothelial cells. With the development of laser vision correction procedures, the RK procedure has been abandoned. However, RK had ramifications for the eventual adoption of PRK and LASIK due to its refractive instability at altitude. Patients who had received RK were eligible for a waiver by the Federal Aviation Administration (FAA), but this procedure has never been approved for military aviation. Prior to the FDA approval of PRK, there were over 1900 civil airmen with RK as of 1994 [37].

Photorefractive Keratectomy

Photorefractive keratectomy, or simply PRK, is a surgical procedure in which an excimer laser under computer control removes a lenticule of stromal tissue resulting in a permanent refractive change, thus allowing for the correction of myopia, hyperopia, and astigmatism. The excimer laser, a 193-nm ultraviolet energy beam, produces a photochemical disruption of molecular bonds. During PRK, the corneal epithelium is typically removed mechanically with a brush, and the excimer laser treatment is then applied to the exposed cornea. Ablation algorithms for conventional treatments are determined by the Munnerlyn formula. The epithelial defect resolves in most cases by 48 h and is typically completely healed within 4–5 days, though the refractive properties and ocular surface abnormalities continues to heal for some time thereafter. Vision considerably improves within 3–4 days following surgery, with correction stabilizing within 3–6 months.

Closely related to PRK is laser epithelial keratomileusis (LASEK), also known as epithelial-LASIK, E-LASIK, or Epi-LASIK. In this variant, a thin flap consisting of just epithelium is carefully separated from the underlying stroma at a hinge for ablation and then reseated following treatment. This variant was developed to potentially mitigate some of the pain and short-term visual disruption that patients can experience after PRK, although many studies have shown no significant advantage when compared to simply removing the epithelium.

Early community studies of conventional PRK treatments on myopic patients were concerning for corneal haze and visual symptoms of haze, glare, or halo, particularly under mesopic conditions [41]. Crucial to the evolution of PRK for use in aviators were efforts to assess the risk of these unfavorable symptoms, and weigh the potential benefits of surgery with the potential loss of an aviator to poor visual outcomes. With study, it was determined that these symptoms were relatively common in the early postoperative period, but tended to resolve by 6 months to 1 year [11]. The use of larger optical zones was noted to reduce visual symptoms [18]. Postoperative refractive predictability was improved over RK but could still result in over or under correction. Fine-tuning of treatment algorithms, smoother ablation profiles, and increased surgeon experience contributed to improved refractive outcomes and patient satisfaction.

After several years of community study, in 1993 the US Navy began investigating the role of PRK in the military. The first study was sponsored by the Special

Warfare Command (Sea, Air, Land team or SEALs), who eventually embraced the procedure as a way to reduce dependence on corrective lenses – an operational necessity for these service members. Thirty myopic active duty Navy and Marine personnel (−2.00 D to −5.50 D, ≤1 D astigmatism) were treated with the Summit OmniMed excimer laser and found no loss of BCVA, with all treated eyes reaching 20/20 UCVA (uncorrected visual acuity) [50]. Glare testing (contrast acuity and intraocular light scatter) was studied noted to return to preoperative levels by 12 months after surgery. Additional PRK studies evaluated mesopic, low-contrast acuity which also showed a return to baseline after surgery. With these early investigations, it was clear that PRK had potential to safely reduce dependence on corrective lenses in military personnel. However, there were several barriers to refractive surgery in aircrew personnel: quality of vision after surgery needed more extensive investigation, and, based on the experience of RK, there were justifiable concerns about refractive stability in hypoxic, hypobaric conditions.

Ongoing with the evolution of PRK were efforts to identify alternative metrics of optical performance in aviators beyond high-contrast Snellen acuity [60]. The limitations of high-contrast acuity testing is well known, especially since vision in flight involves low-light and low-contrast conditions. Two tests in particular were shown to be of value: low-contrast acuity and low-light low-contrast acuity. This is particularly important in aviators; for instance, night carrier operations are widely regarded as the single most challenging and visually demanding task an aviator must complete (Fig. 3.2). As such, visual quality and, in particular, low-contrast acuity were

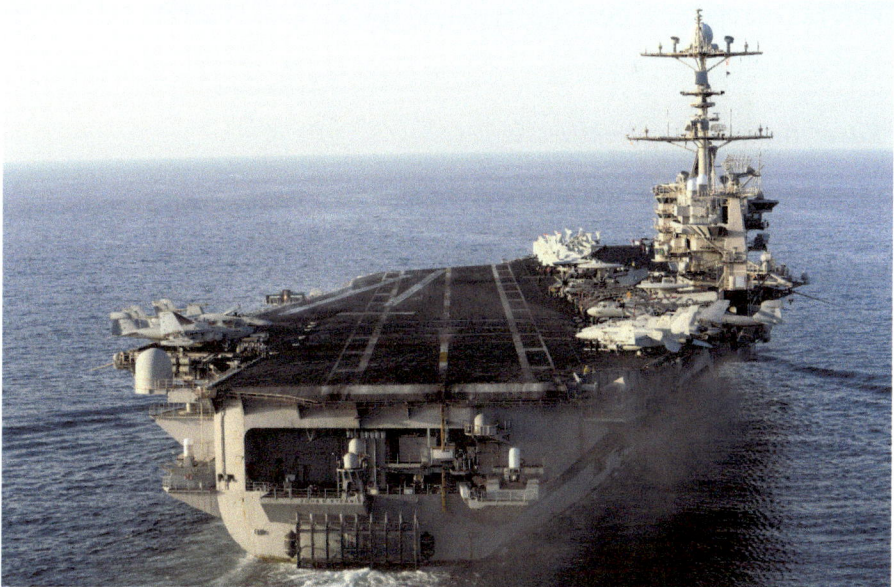

Fig. 3.2 Carrier landing operations pose a demanding visual task, particularly in low-light conditions

closely followed in early trials with the foresight toward the use of refractive procedures in aviators. Ongoing study of PRK on non-aircrew military personnel reassuringly supported that mean mesopic acuity was as good as or better than preoperative performance after surgery [50].

Refractive stability at altitude was one of the key areas of interest prior to approval. PRK was studied alongside RK and control myopic patients at the US Army Pikes Peak Research Laboratory (elevation 14,100 ft) [27]. In this study, control myopic eyes and PRK-treated eyes exhibited slight corneal thickening but no change in refractive error at altitude.

Numerous improvements in the PRK procedure during the 1990s resulted in a very low risk for long-term glare disability or reduced contrast sensitivity. In 1999, the US Navy entered into trials permitting PRK to be performed on designated aviators and student aviator applicants, referred to as the "retention" and "accessions" studies. In the "accessions" study, 300 PRK patients entered flight training and were compared to over 4000 controls [53]. The PRK-treated patients had a lower attrition rate and performed as well as or better than their counterparts in academics and flight performance in all study metrics. Following the results of this study, new applicants were allowed to receive waivers for PRK in order to meet visual requirements.

As part of the "Retention of Naval Aviators PRK Study," 785 aviators (150 pilots and 635 aircrew) received PRK between 2000 and 2005 [53]. In this study, 90% of aviators were eligible to return to flight duty without correction by 6 weeks. No aviator suffered visual complications precluding flight duty. The results of this study supported the role of PRK in designated aviators. With the results of these studies, PRK became approved for waiver in civil airmen and military aviators.

Laser In Situ Keratomileusis

In the wake of the success with the adoption of PRK, attention shifted to laser in situ keratomileusis, or LASIK, a form of corneal refractive procedure which involves the creation of a flap in the corneal stroma, leaving the epithelium intact. After flap creation using a mechanical microkeratome or a femtosecond laser, the corneal flap is folded away from the ablation bed and the excimer laser then applied to the exposed stroma to reshape and treat refractive errors (Fig. 3.3). Following ablation, the flap is reseated and allowed to heal. Most patients experience prompt uncorrected visual improvement, and the visual recovery after LASIK is much faster than PRK. This is an attractive option for aviators as it substantially reduces postoperative downtime. However, similar to PRK, rigorous clinical evaluation was needed before the procedure could be given the green light in aircrew. In the movement toward LASIK, emphasis was placed not only on the quality of visual outcomes but also on the integrity of the corneal flap.

Early retrospective comparisons of conventional PRK and LASIK on non-aircrew personnel suggested that LASIK eyes experienced a mean loss of contrast acuity after surgery, which did not fully resolve over the follow-up time period [9].

Fig. 3.3 Surgeon's view during excimer laser ablation. In this LASIK procedure, the flap has been created and folded away from the ablation bed (Courtesy of SC Schallhorn)

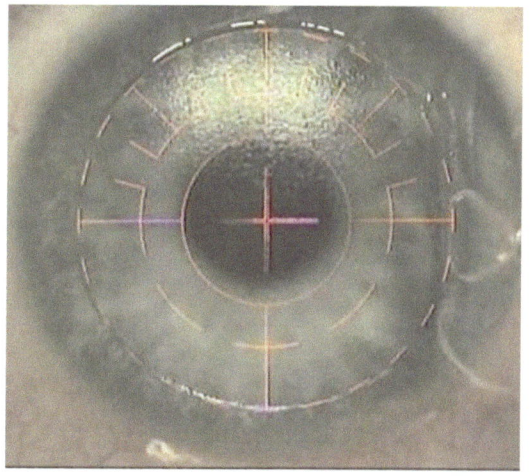

In this same study, PRK patients tended to experience fewer symptoms of glare and halo than LASIK. Study of night driving simulator performance on recipients of conventional LASIK revealed a decrease both in target detection and target identification distance after surgery, with and without a glare source. Conventional LASIK, performed with the use of microkeratome for flap creation and standard ablation algorithms, was not ready for aircrew in its early stages.

Several technological advances would occur that would pave the way for the ultimate study and approval of LASIK in aircrew. Notably, the paring of wavefront-guided (WFG) and femtosecond technologies would prove to be the pivotal step in optimizing visual outcomes (Fig. 3.4). Evidence had been accumulating that WFG technology offered the ability to correct optical aberrations, resulting in improved contrast sensitivity [22]. A matched dataset comparison of conventional LASIK and PRK with WFG LASIK provided supportive evidence that WFG treatments produce more predictable refractive outcomes than conventional treatments, with improved best corrected and low-contrast visual acuity [48]. Femtosecond-assisted LASIK had been independently evaluated in numerous studies on non-aviators and demonstrated to be safe and efficacious in the creation of flaps for the treatment of refractive error [12].

In the setting of building evidence supporting the role of these new technologies, direct comparison of mechanical microkeratome and femtosecond-assisted WFG LASIK in military personnel demonstrated faster visual recovery in the femtosecond group, with a higher percentage of eyes reaching uncorrected acuity of 20/16 or greater [57]. Comparison of night driving performance after conventional and WFG femtosecond-assisted LASIK demonstrated significantly improved mean night driving visual performance [51]. The results of this study were instrumental in the decision to allow LASIK to become acceptable for civilian and military aviators, including astronauts.

Currently, all forms of LASIK and PRK are eligible for waiver for aviators in any role in civilian or military aviation. Formal approval of CRS in civilian aviators

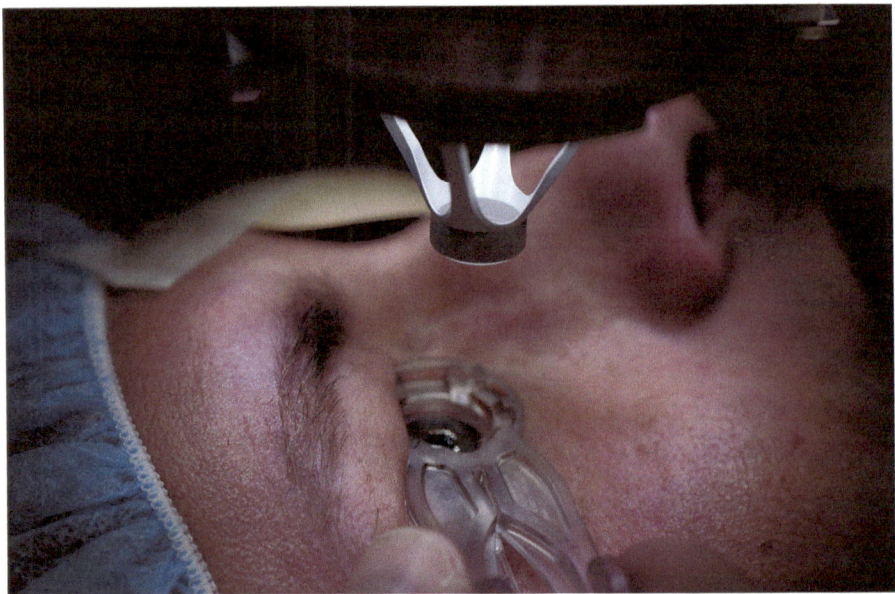

Fig. 3.4 Patient interface for LASIK flap creation using femtosecond laser technology. In this image, a specialized suction device is applied to the eye, designed to dock with the femtosecond laser for applanation of the cornea during flap creation (Courtesy of SC Schallhorn)

occurred in 2004. US Army pilots were eligible for waiver following the introduction of the Army Warfighter Refractive Eye Surgery Program, which was initiated in 2000. Waivers for PRK in US Air Force pilots and aircrew began being granted in 2000. Air Force aircrew received approval for LASIK in 2007. Approval of PRK in US Navy aviators and applicants first occurred in 2004, following the results of the "accessions" and "retentions" studies. Routine waiver recommendations for designated Naval aviators and aircrew for LASIK occurred in 2012 and for student applicants in 2013. LASIK was also approved for use in astronauts in June, 2007. Presently, one current qualified astronaut has received LASIK, and in the most recent applicant cycle, several applicants were noted to have received some form of laser vision correction.

Current Policies and Procedures

Refractive Surgery Techniques - Advanced Ablation Profiles

Wavefront-guided technology enables the measurement and quantification of lower- and higher-order optical aberrations through the methods of wavefront mapping. By convention, a clinical refraction, which is used to guide refractive surgery treatments, is composed of sphere, cylinder, and axis: the so called lower-order aberrations. Coma and spherical aberration are common types of higher-order optical aberrations (HOA) which cannot be identified on a routine clinical evaluation, but can contribute to image blur and visual symptoms.

Two advanced ablation profiles have been developed to minimize HOA: (a) wavefront-guided (WFG) ablation, which creates a profile based on all ocular aberrations as measured by an aberrometer device, and (b) wavefront-optimized (WFO) ablation, which creates a profile based on the manifest refraction and is adjusted to reduce the induction of spherical aberration. These advanced ablation techniques have been independently evaluated in both PRK and LASIK. Spherical aberration can be significantly increased after a myopic conventional ablation profile, and both WFG and WFO procedures result in less induction (or reduction) of spherical aberration with resulting improvement in visual quality [52].

Current recommendations for refractive surgery in aviators favor use of an advanced ablation algorithm. Military refractive surgeons routinely perform procedures with these technologies on active duty service members, including aircrew, reverting to conventional ablation algorithms only in rare circumstances.

Visual Outcomes of Corneal Refractive Surgery in Aviators

After the approval of laser vision correction in civilian and military aviation communities, a wealth of knowledge has been generated underscoring the safety and efficacy of PRK and LASIK procedures across a variety of environments. The study of LASIK in US Naval aviators demonstrated the safety of WFG femtosecond LASIK in aircrew with duties involving actual control of aircraft [56]. In this trial, 548 eyes with myopia, 60 eyes with mixed astigmatism, and 25 eyes with hyperopia underwent WFG femtosecond LASIK. Uncorrected acuity of 20/20 was reached in 98.3% of myopic/astigmatic eyes and 95.7% of hyperopic eyes, with almost all eyes maintaining spherical equivalent (SE) within ±1.00 D postoperatively. Low-contrast acuity (25% level) was improved in more than 40% of eyes in all groups. A subtle but statistically significant increase in HOAs was observed (root mean square +0.03 ± 0.10 μm standard deviation).

In a prospective study on 20 US Army UH-60 Black Hawk pilots, 22 eyes received PRK and 18 eyes received LASIK [62]. At 1 month after surgery, 10 of 11 PRK patients were able to meet visual acuity standards to return to duty. One PRK patient had persistent corneal haze, which resolved at 3 months at which point he was able to return to flight status.

In a study on Air Force pilots in the Republic of Korea following the approval of CRS in 2007, 38 eyes of 20 subjects underwent PRK and were followed for 4 years postoperatively [32]. In this cohort, 89.5% of eyes reached UCVA of 20/20 or better, with no eyes losing any line of best corrected acuity. Refractions were stable at 4 years despite high-altitude environmental exposure.

Safety

To date there have been no aviation mishaps directly attributed to complications following refractive surgery. There has been one report of a designated pilot being permanently taken off of flight status after PRK [10]. During the early postoperative period following uneventful PRK, a 46-year-old male C-130 senior pilot was placed on topical steroids for treatment of corneal inflammation and scarring. On postoperative day 24, the patient presented for evaluation with complaint of decreased vision and ocular pain. He was found to have ocular hypertension which necessitated treatment with topical glaucoma medications. A non-arteritic anterior ischemic optic neuropathy was observed by postoperative day 29. On follow-up evaluation approximately 9 months after onset of symptoms, he was found to have severe visual field constriction in the affected eye with a best corrected acuity of 20/50, resulting in removal from flight status.

Altitude and Hypoxia

There have been a number of reports and evaluations of both PRK and LASIK in hypobaric and hypoxic environments. As previously discussed, in study atop the US Army Pikes Peak Research Laboratory at 14,100 ft, PRK-treated eyes exhibited slight corneal thickening but no change in refractive error [27].

In 2001, a published report described a temporary, reversible myopic shift with resulting loss of distance visual acuity in two climbers during an ascent to nearly 23,000 ft. Both climbers had previously received uneventful myopic LASIK [4].

The effect of ambient hypoxia and low humidity was studied on active duty LASIK patients by Larys and Schallhorn (unpublished data) using modified goggles [Reduced Oxygen Delivery Device (RODD), Environics, Hartford, Connecticut, USA]. In this study simulating conditions of a nonpressurized V-22 Osprey aircraft at 25,000 ft, eyes were randomized to dry air or low humidity for 2.5 h. No significant changes in refraction, uncorrected acuity, or contrast sensitivity were observed. Study of exposure to hypoxic conditions simulating an altitude of 35,000 ft similarly revealed no significant changes to corneal curvature, refractive error, or visual performance on post-LASIK subjects [1].

PRK and LASIK Topics

Minimizing Risk of Corneal Haze

Corneal haze is a well-recognized complication of PRK, and is particularly of concern to the aviator given its potential to degrade quality of vision. Haze is developed from subepithelial scarring following ablation and can lead to irregular astigmatism and loss of UCVA. Modern WFG PRK procedures and ablation techniques are the result of a myriad of trials investigating methods to improve postoperative acuity and mitigate undesirable visual symptoms including the development of haze. The risk appears to correlate with the amount of tissue ablation [44], such that highly myopic patients are at relatively increased risk. The prophylactic application of the alkylating agent mitomycin C applied to the ablated corneal stroma following PRK reduces the risk of postoperative haze [61]. This technique, while surgeon dependent, has become relatively widespread in use, including pilots and aircrew.

Flap Stability

Following approval, ongoing efforts have been underway to evaluate flap integrity and visual stability under stresses of hypoxic and hypobaric conditions. Complications such as flap displacement or slip, if elicited by forces of acceleration, wind blast, rapid decompression, or other flight-related turbulence would potentially be catastrophic. Study of the LASIK flap in simulated aircraft ejection environments in rabbit models provided the groundwork supporting good flap integrity to extreme windblast forces simulating ejection [16]. Biomechanical studies of the flap revealed a significant wind blast force required to cause flap dislocation [25], and these forces are greater in femtosecond-created flaps when compared to microkeratome flaps [23].

The risk of flap displacement after LASIK has been studied in a large retrospective case series and found to be very low (0.012%) [8]. In this study, all flap displacements occurred within 48 h of surgery and were not preceded by ocular trauma. The risk, while exceedingly low, may be higher following hyperopic treatments or use of microkeratome for flap creation.

There has been a report of a late traumatic flap displacement after LASIK in one activity duty service member, unrelated to aviation duties [14]. This individual experienced flap displacement following blunt trauma to the operative eye 2 months after LASIK, but prompt identification of this vision-threatening injury and transfer to a specialist allowed visual recovery to 20/20 uncorrected by as early as 7 days following the injury.

Femtosecond LASIK

As a class, the advantages of femtosecond devices over microkeratome to create flaps for refractive procedures are numerous. Femtosecond lasers reliably generate accurate and precise flaps of programmable diameter and thickness, allowing for the tailoring of flap size to ablation zone. The flaps are planar in morphology, as opposed to the meniscus shaped flaps of the microkeratome, which are thicker at the edges. The side-cut angle is often customizable (Fig. 3.5), which can assist with proper flap

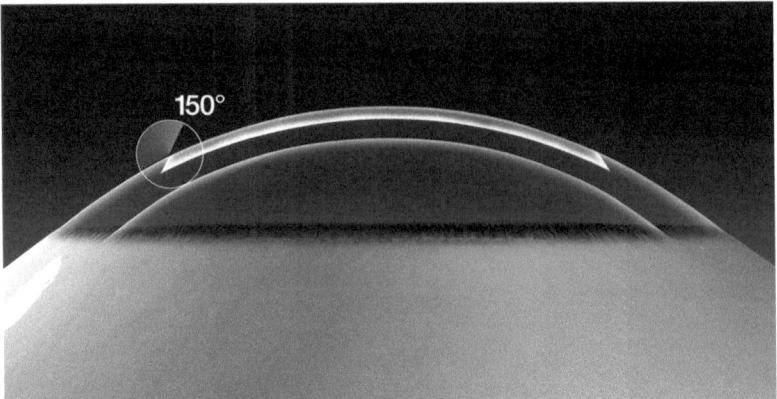

Fig. 3.5 Side-cut angle is a parameter uniquely customizable by many femtosecond platforms. The side-cut angle can be inverted (>90°), whereby the flap margin can be tucked under the adjacent tissue, promoting proper alignment and seating (Courtesy of Abbott Medical Optics, Inc., Santa Ana, CA)

seating postoperatively and may reduce risk of flap dislocation. Lastly, femtosecond flaps tend to create a robust healing response in the peripheral side cut that has been associated with improved flap adhesion over a microkeratome created flap [23]. Side-cut angle is important to consider in flap adhesion, as inverted side cuts tuck the cut flap edge under adjacent stroma, providing a barrier to dislocation and reducing risk for epithelial ingrowth [24].

Femtosecond-assisted WFG LASIK is considered safe and efficacious in the treatment of refractive error and may facilitate faster visual recovery and a higher proportion of treated eyes reaching uncorrected acuity of 20/16 or better. Large retrospective study published following the approval in civil airmen provided further evidence supporting outcomes of femtosecond-assisted LASIK [55]. However, femtosecond LASIK has its own unique complications, such as rainbow glare and transient light sensitivity syndrome [3, 33], which could pose potential hazards for aviation personnel. The incidence of rainbow glare and transient light sensitivity syndrome are rare, and if it occurs in aviators or aircrew, they should not be flying until it resolves to minimize distractions.

Military-Specific Topics

Ejection

For military aviation, refractive surgery has historically been controversial due to concerns about corneal safety and stability in ejection scenarios. There have been reports supporting the safety of PRK-operated eyes even in these environments which reassuringly supports the role of PRK in military communities [58]. For instance, the case of one aviator, 6 months out from PRK, ejected from a Navy S-3B Viking aircraft while performing field carrier landing practice. There were no visual consequences of the ejection, and follow-up examination demonstrated stable visual acuity. The mishap was unrelated to visual function or surgery. More recently, there has emerged a report of a male F/A-18F Super Hornet naval flight officer who ejected at 13,000 feet at speeds greater than 350 knots. The aviator had received LASIK 7 years prior, and following ejection, no flap related complications or defects were identified, with BCVA of 20/15 in both eyes [66].

Additional Refractive Procedures and Related Topics

Femtosecond Lenticular Extraction

A new technique has been developed which utilizes a femtosecond laser to correct myopia (without the need for an excimer laser), also called the small incision lenticule extraction (SMILE). The technique involves using a femtosecond laser to cut a precisely defined lenticule at mid-stromal depth which is then removed through a side incision. The VisuMax Femtosecond Laser (Carl Zeiss Meditec, Dublin, CA) is currently the only femtosecond platform that has received FDA approval to perform the SMILE procedure for the correction of myopia [67]. Outside of the United States, approximately 700,000 procedures have been performed.

SMILE has potential advantages over PRK and LASIK for aviators. A recently conducted meta-analysis of 11 peer-reviewed studies which compared femtosecond lenticular extraction to femtosecond LASIK concluded that both procedures had comparable safety and efficacy in terms of refractive and visual outcomes and change in best corrected vision [65]. The femtosecond lenticular removal may result in fewer dry eye symptoms and less loss of postoperative corneal sensitivity. There are also reported biomechanical advantages that may make the cornea more stable and resistant to trauma [46]. SMILE could reduce or eliminated certain LASIK flap complications, such as traumatic flap dislocation. In addition, the visual recovery should be significantly faster than PRK. Surveillance of visual outcomes by aviation communities will be needed to monitor for safety of this procedure in aviators and aircrew.

Intrastromal Corneal Ring Segments

Intrastromal corneal ring segments (ICRSs) are FDA approved for the treatment of myopia. These are small devices made of PMMA (polymethyl methacrylate) which are implanted in the deep corneal stroma to modify the corneal curvature. Civil airmen who have received the procedure may be eligible for waiver provided they meet all visual standards. This procedure is not approved for military aviators.

Phakic Intraocular Lens/Implantable Collamer Lens

Phakic intraocular lenses (pIOLs), also referred to as implantable collamer lenses (ICLs), are artificial intraocular lenses used for the treatment of myopia. Two lenses of this class are currently FDA approved: one iris fixated in the anterior chamber and one placed in the posterior chamber. A broad range of refractive errors can safely be treated, with rapid visual recovery and stable refraction [49]. The procedure is a viable alternative for patients who are not good candidates for laser vision correction, such as those with dry eye disease, inadequate corneal stroma, or high levels of refractive error. Risks include endothelial cell loss, cataract formation, secondary glaucoma, iris atrophy, and traumatic lens dislocation [19]. The procedure has not received dedicated evaluation by aviation communities. Civil airmen who have received this procedure are eligible for waiver. The procedure is currently considered disqualifying for military aviators, though waivers may soon be considered for non-pilots and aircrew.

Refractive Lens Exchange

Refractive lens exchange (RLE) involves the removal of the clear natural lens and replacement with an implant; similar to cataract surgery, however, the procedure is performed without cataract formation. In this case, the indications are strictly refractive, with the procedure being offered to patients who would otherwise not be a candidate for laser vision correction, such as those with very high levels of refractive error. Hyperopia, myopia, and mixed astigmatism may be treated with RLE. As the procedure involves removal of the natural lens, accommodative abilities are lost after surgery. Refractive lens exchange outcomes are less published and have not been evaluated in aviation communities. Notable risks include retinal detachment, which may be as high as 8% in highly myopic patients, and posterior capsule opacification (PCO). The procedure is approved for civil airmen provided all vision standards are met. The procedure is considered disqualifying for military aviators. Waivers are considered for non-pilots and aircrew on a case by case basis provided vision standards and refractive standards are met, and there are no concerning complications which may interfere with duties involving flying.

Presbyopia and Monovision

Presbyopia, the progressive loss of lens accommodation with age, is a common issue in aviators over the age of 40. Currently there are a multitude of therapies available for the treatment of this condition, most commonly corrective lenses in the form of bifocal spectacles or contact lenses. Multifocal contact lenses are FAA approved in civil aircrew, subject to a 1-month wait to allow for adaptation before returning to aviation duties. Monovision with contact lenses is not approved, as there have been concerns related to safety with this method after an airline accident was attributed to altered visual perception secondary to contact lens monovision [36].

There are select surgical options that have been utilized in the treatment of presbyopia, to varying degrees of success. In the realm of aviation, however, these surgical options have not been thoroughly evaluated. Most surgical corrections for presbyopia entail monovision, wherein one eye is corrected for distant vision and the fellow eye for near vision. In this type of procedure, stereopsis can be compromised. Currently, no surgical treatment of presbyopia has been approved for use in military aviation.

Laser Vision Presbyopia Correction

Laser vision correction has been utilized for the treatment of presbyopia, principally involving treatment with monovision. There are cases of surgical monovision being performed safely in aviators dating back to 1997 [29]. Surgical monovision is conditionally approved for select civil aircrew following a mandatory postoperative waiting period of 6 months to allow for adaptation and completion of a medical flight test. There have not been large-scale studies to evaluate the safety of this modality in aircrew, though the use of contact lenses to achieve similar monovision effects has been identified as causal to at least one aviation mishap [36].

Corneal Inlays and Presbyopia

Two types of corneal inlays are now FDA approved for the treatment of presbyopia. Corneal inlays function to overcome the inability of the natural lens to accommodate. They may be surgically implanted into the anterior corneal stroma in either a LASIK flap or corneal pocket. Principally, there are three categories of inlays: refractive optics, corneal reshaping, and small aperture [26]. Refractive optical inlays utilize special materials to create a central area for distant vision, surrounded by one or more rings to add refractive power for near vision. Corneal reshaping implants modulate the anterior curvature of the corneal to enhance near and intermediate vision. Small-aperture inlays function like a pinhole to limit incident light rays to those parallel with the visual axis, thus minimizing the need for refraction and allowing for simultaneous near and distant vision. There is no official policy on these procedures for civilian aviation and they are not approved for military aviators.

Laser Thermal Keratoplasty and Conductive Keratoplasty to Treat Presbyopia

Laser thermal keratoplasty (LTK) and conductive keratoplasty (CK) are noninvasive refractive procedures to treat presbyopia or low levels of hyperopia. In these two similar procedures, thermal energy is applied to the peripheral cornea, which heats and shrinks collagen fibrils, resulting in increased curvature of the central cornea and increased refractive power. In LTK this energy is supplied via a holmium/YAG laser; in CK a keratoplast tip is inserted and radiofrequency current is applied. These procedures have more or less been abandoned today. They have been previously been studied in non-aviators and found to be safe and efficacious [30, 31]. Both procedures are considered temporary, as the amount of correction will decrease over time. CK has also been studied in the treatment of hyperopic overcorrection of myopic eyes after LASIK [6]. Civilian patients who have received this procedure are eligible for a waiver, provided at least 6 months has elapsed following surgery to allow for adaptation. A medical flight test may be necessary. This procedure is considered disqualifying for military aviation personnel.

Cataract Surgery and Aviators

Of special mention in the discussion of refractive surgery in aviators is the topic of the development of cataracts and the cataract removal surgery. Cataract formation in the lens of the eye is the end result of complex, multifactorial, and incompletely understood processes [21]. Replacement of an opaque cataract with a synthetic lens has origins tied with the aviation community [2]. Sir Harold Ridley was the first to note that aviators during World War II had insignificant and visually inert responses to foreign body fragments of aircraft canopies that had traumatically entered the eye. Canopies of the era were made of glass or PMMA (also known as 'Plexiglas'), the latter of which would prove to be the material of choice for early intraocular lens operations.

Visually significant cataracts are considered disqualifying for aviators in any role, given the symptoms of glare and reduced acuity can be significant safety concerns for night operations. Aircrew have successfully received cataract surgery and returned to aviation duty dating back to the 1980s. A number of reports have emerged detailing the safety of aphakic or pseudophakic patients in civilian aviation roles [34]. Stability of the intraocular lens (IOL) in flight has been documented in military communities [20] and even one report in an astronaut with bilateral IOLs [28].

Visual disturbances related to cataract progression are typically problems of the aging aviator. Visually significant cataracts, manifest by decreased visual acuity out of required standards, positive glare test, or debilitating symptoms, are considered disqualifying for all aviators. However, provided the patient meets visual acuity standards postoperatively, cataract surgery requires no waiver from the FAA. There is a mandatory 3-month wait for multifocal or accommodative lens implants after surgery to allow for adaptation. Waivers may be issued for military aircrew on a case by case basis.

Evidence has accumulated over time that aircrew, and indeed astronauts, are at higher risk for cataracts and tend to present at a younger age. The extent to which aircrew are at increased susceptibility to this common, age-related condition has been difficult to quantify. In a population-based case-control study of 445 men, the odds ratio for nuclear cataract for pilots compared with non-pilots was 3.02 (95% confidence interval 1.44–6.35), adjusted for age, smoking status, and sunbathing habits. The etiology of this increased cataract risk has been difficult to attribute to interaction with the flight environment, with specific considerations directed toward increased radiation exposure associated with high altitudes. Incidence may be highest in astronauts [45].

In a study exploring the mechanisms of cataract in US Air Force and Navy aviators as well as astronauts, aviators tended to develop subcapsular cataracts, in comparison to cortical cataracts in astronauts [21]. The increased risk in aviators may be associated with various forms of occupational radiation exposure, such as UV and gamma radiation. In astronauts, there is interest in further understanding the effects of cosmic radiation exposure and cataracts, with studies demonstrating some degree of association between severity of cortical opacity and radiation [7].

Waiver Process for Refractive Surgery

Currently, all forms of PRK and LASIK are considered disqualifying for aviation for civilian and military pilots and aircrew, though waivers are routinely granted for these procedures. Eligibility for CRS among aircrew correlates with prevalence of ametropia and corrective lens use. In a retrospective review of US Air Force pilots from 1999 to 2008, among 12,951 pilots, 41% (5312) required corrective lens use for flight duty [64]. An estimated 2731 of these pilots would meet cycloplegic refraction criteria for CRS. At time of writing, an estimated 7.0% of these eligible pilots had received CRS.

PRK remains the preferred form of refractive surgery, including in aviators, primarily due to patient preference. The Naval Aerospace Medical Institute (NAMI) staff routinely encourage LASIK over PRK for aviation personell and civilian applicants to avoid potential complications of corneal haze, but final decision rests with the patient and surgeon. The Naval Aeromedical Reference and Waiver Guide states that WFG femtosecond LASIK is the preferred treatment of choice for designated aviators and applicants.

Civil Aviators

Regardless of specific roles or community, the general policies outlining CRS are to maintain acceptable levels of safety. For civil airmen, the FAA requires that airmen with refractive surgical procedures by removed from flying duties until adequate healing has taken place, vision is stable, and no significant adverse effects or complications have occurred [43]. For most refractive procedures, including PRK and LASIK, aviators may return to duty with their valid medical certificate under 14 Code of Federal Regulations section 61.53 as soon as the eye care provider gives authorization and appropriate visual acuity standards are met. A report of eye evaluation (FAA Form 8500-7) will need to be completed by the eye care provider and provided to the aviation medical examiner (AME) at the next scheduled FAA medical examination. This report should detail that appropriate postoperative healing has taken place, visual acuity is stable, and there are no complications or residual debilitating symptoms, such as glare, haze, or halos. Once this report has been documented at the next AME visit, special issuance of a medical certificate may be granted. The report may also be submitted to the FAA Office of Aerospace Medicine, stating:

> (T)he airman meets the visual acuity standards and the report of eye evaluation indicates healing is complete, visual acuity remains stable, and the applicant does not suffer sequela, such as glare intolerance, halos, rings, impaired night vision, or any other complications.

Airmen are able to pursue refractive procedures on their own capacity, with online educational resources supplied by the FAA [38]. Online guides are available for aviation medical examiners [17].

Refractive monovision is approved in civil airmen, with additional regulatory precautions. For medical certification, a 6-month adaptation period is mandatory. During this waiting period, corrective lenses may be used to meet visual acuity standards for both eyes. At the completion of the 6-month waiting period, a medical flight test authorized by the FAA Aerospace Medical Certification Division is necessary. After successful completion of the medical flight test, a Statement of Demonstrated Ability may be issued. In additional circumstances where there may be concern for quality and function of vision, not restricted to monovision, a medical flight test may also be performed.

Military Pilots and Aircrew

For current and prospective military aviators, current policy dictates that laser vision correction procedures are considered disqualifying for aviation duties, however these policies are in flux and may be subject to change. PRK and LASIK are routinely eligible for waiver, depending on pre-operative refraction, with distinct guidelines for active duty aviators and new applicants. Designated aviators and aircrew are eligible to pursue refractive surgery at Department of Defense centers provided they are good candidates for the procedure and receive command approval. Civilian applicants may receive the procedure on their own expense in order to meet vision standards. There are currently limits on refractive correction that impact waiver eligibility, which vary for designated pilots, aircrew, and applicants.

Civilian Student Naval Aviator applicants are limited to +3.00D to −8.00D of sphere, 3D of cylinder, and 3.50D of anisometropia with a six-month wait time prior to military entrance; civilian non-aviator applicants may have pre-op hyperopia up to +6.00D of sphere, all other parameters being equal. Designated naval aviation personnel may have any pre-op refraction prior to PRK, and for LASIK +6.00D to −11.5D sphere pre-operatively. US Air Force and US Army standards are similar.

The waiver process for designated aviators and aircrew is initiated after they have received surgery. Mandatory postoperative recovery time before waiver eligibility will vary by procedure (PRK or LASIK) and the type and level of refractive treatment administered. As an example, current wait times for designated naval aviators are as follows:

1. *A PRK waiver request may be submitted after the following wait periods:*

   (a) *Myopia −6.00 diopters or less spherical equivalent (SE): 3 months*
   (b) *Myopia greater than −6.00 diopters SE: 6 months*
   (c) *Hyperopia SE: 6 months*

2. *A LASIK waiver request may be submitted after the following wait periods:*

   (d) *Myopia correction up to −11.5D SE: 2 weeks*
   (e) *Hyperopia up to + 4D SE: 4 weeks*
   (f) *Hyperopia greater than +4D SE and up to +6D SE: 8 weeks*

Once the mandatory recovery period has elapsed, the service member will report to their local eye care provider. A vision questionnaire will be completed to ensure the absence of debilitating visual symptoms such as glare or halos. Once the eye care provider has determined that healing has completed, there are no adverse postoperative symptoms, and the patient meets all vision standards for their class, recommendation for return to full duty will be forwarded to the flight surgeon. The flight surgeon will perform a complete examination to ensure there are no other adverse sequelae. An "Aeromedical Summary" (AMS) may then be completed by the flight surgeon or eye care provider. The AMS details the patient's flight role, preoperative and postoperative examination, operative reports, and any residual symptoms or findings which may impact return to aviation duty. Reports from the flight physical examination and AMS will be forwarded to NAMI for review by an Aerospace Ophthalmologist or Aerospace Optometrist. If deemed warranted, NAMI will then make a recommendation for waiver to the Bureau of Personnel (Navy) or Commandant of the Marine Corps (US Marine Corps), who will make the ultimate determination to issue the waiver for return to flight duty.

Final Thoughts

The advent of corneal refractive surgery into the realm of aviation has been the focus of extensive research over the last several decades. The aviation environment is filled with noxious ocular stimuli, including hypoxia, hypobaria, low humidity, and circulating particulate matter. Spectacles and contact lenses remain the most

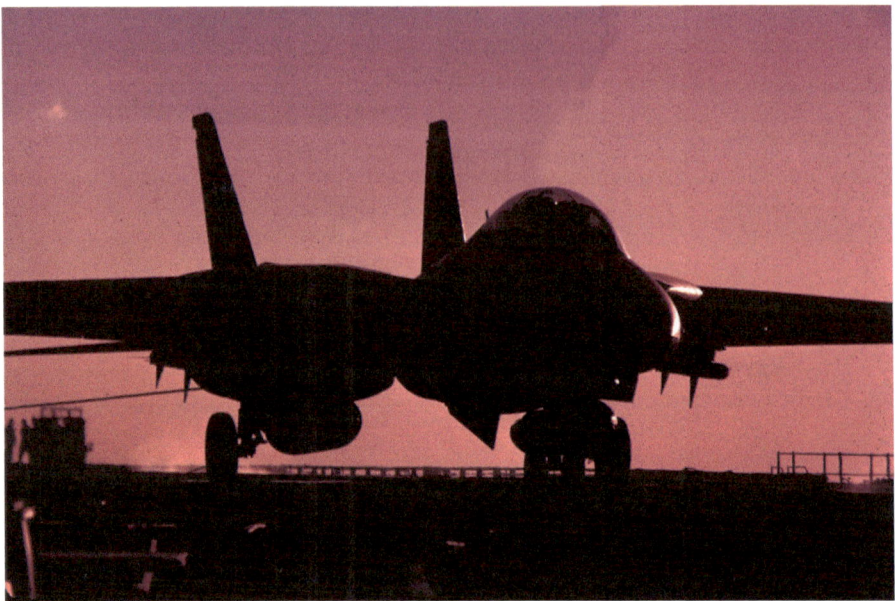

Fig. 3.6 Corneal refractive procedures will continue to play an important role for current and future generations of aviators

common form of vision correction utilized, but can be ill suited to turbulent forces or incompatible with modern avionics equipment. The refractive procedures PRK and LASIK are safe and efficacious methods to reduce dependence on corrective lens use and have been well validated in a number of aviation communities. SMILE may represent the future of refractive surgery in pilots and aircrew. Refractive procedures have and will continue to play an important role for current and future generations of aviation crewmen (Fig. 3.6).

Compliance with Ethical Requirements
Craig S. Schallhorn, M.D. has no conflict of interest.
Steve C. Schallhorn, M.D. is Chief Medical Officer for Carl Zeiss Meditec, Inc.
No human studies were carried out by the authors for this article.
No animal studies were carried out by the authors for this article.

References

1. Aaron M, Wright S, Gooch J, Harvey R, Davis R, Reilly C. Stability of laser-assisted in situ keratomileusis (LASIK) at altitude. Aviat Space Environ Med. 2012;83(10):958–61. doi:10.3357/asem.3325.2012.
2. Apple DJ, Sims J. Harold Ridley and the invention of the intraocular lens. Surv Ophthalmol. 1996;40(4):279–92.

3. Bamba S, Rocha KM, Ramos-Esteban JC, Krueger RR. Incidence of rainbow glare after laser in situ keratomileusis flap creation with a 60 kHz femtosecond laser. J Cataract Refract Surg. 2009;35(6):1082–6. doi:10.1016/j.jcrs.2009.01.026.

4. Boes DA, Omura AK, Hennessy MJ. Effect of high-altitude exposure on myopic laser in situ keratomileusis. J Cataract Refract Surg. 2001;27(12):1937–41.

5. Capó-Aponte JE, Hilber DJ, Urosevich TG, Lattimore MR, Weaver JL. Military aircrew eyewear survey: operational issues. Aviat Space Environ Med. 2013;84(8):814–22. doi:10.3357/asem.3514.2013.

6. Chang JS, Lau SY. Conductive keratoplasty to treat hyperopic overcorrection after LASIK for myopia. J Refract Surg. 2011;27(1):49–55. doi:10.3928/1081597X-20100212-10.

7. Chylack LT Jr, Peterson LE, Feiveson AH, Wear ML, Manuel FK, Tung WH, Hardy DS, Marak LJ, Cucinotta FA. NASA study of cataract in astronauts (NASCA). Report 1: cross-sectional study of the relationship of exposure to space radiation and risk of lens opacity. Radiat Res. 2009;172(1):10–20. doi:10.1667/RR1580.1.

8. Clare G, Moore TC, Grills C, Leccisotti A, Moore JE, Schallhorn S. Early flap displacement after LASIK. Ophthalmology. 2011;118(9):1760–5. doi:10.1016/j.ophtha.2011.01.053.

9. Dalton M (2007) LASIK with IntraLase now being studied in aviators.

10. Davis RE, Ivan DJ, Rubin RM, Gooch JM, Tredici TJ, Reilly CD. Permanent grounding of a USAF pilot following photorefractive keratectomy. Aviat Space Environ Med. 2010;81(11):1041–4.

11. Fan-Paul NI, Li J, Miller JS, Florakis GJ. Night vision disturbances after corneal refractive surgery. Surv Ophthalmol. 2002;47(6):533–46.

12. Farjo AA, Sugar A, Schallhorn SC, Majmudar PA, Tanzer DJ, Trattler WB, Cason JB, Donaldson KE, Kymionis GD. Femtosecond lasers for LASIK flap creation: a report by the American Academy of Ophthalmology. Ophthalmology. 2013;120(3):e5–e20. doi:10.1016/j.ophtha.2012.08.013.

13. Flynn WJ, Miller RE 2nd, Tredici TJ, Block MG, Kirby EE, Provines WF. Contact lens wear at altitude: subcontact lens bubble formation. Aviat Space Environ Med. 1987;58(11):1115–8.

14. Franklin QJ, Tanzer DJ. Late traumatic flap displacement after laser in situ keratomileuisis. Mil Med. 2004;169(4):334–6.

15. Gibson CR, Mader TH, Schallhorn SC, Pesudovs K, Lipsky W, Raid E, Jennings RT, Fogarty JA, Garriott RA, Garriott OK, Johnston SL. Visual stability of laser vision correction in an astronaut on a Soyuz mission to the International Space Station. J Cataract Refract Surg. 2012;38(8):1486–91. doi:10.1016/j.jcrs.2012.06.012.

16. Goodman RL, Johnson DA, Dillon H, Edelhauser HF, Waller SG. Laser in situ keratomileusis flap stability during simulated aircraft ejection in a rabbit model. Cornea. 2003;22(2):142–5.

17. Guide for Aviation Medical Examiners: items 31–34. Eye – refractive procedures. Federal Aviation Administration. https://www.faa.gov/about/office_org/headquarters_offices/avs/offices/aam/ame/guide/app_process/exam_tech/et/31-34/rp/. Accessed July 2016.

18. Hersh PS, Stulting RD, Steinert RF, Waring GO 3rd, Thompson KP, O'Connell M, Doney K, Schein OD. Results of phase III excimer laser photorefractive keratectomy for myopia. The Summit PRK Study Group. Ophthalmology. 1997;104(10):1535–53.

19. Huang D, Schallhorn SC, Sugar A, Farjo AA, Majmudar PA, Trattler WB, Tanzer DJ. Phakic intraocular lens implantation for the correction of myopia: a report by the American Academy of Ophthalmology. Ophthalmology. 2009;116(11):2244–58. doi:10.1016/j.ophtha.2009.08.018.

20. Ivan DJ, Tredici TJ. Intraocular lenses in military aircrew. Defense Technical Information Center. (2000). http://www.dtic.mil/dtic/tr/fulltext/u2/p010580.pdf.

21. Jones JA, McCarten M, Manuel K, Djojonegoro B, Murray J, Feiversen A, Wear M. Cataract formation mechanisms and risk in aviation and space crews. Aviat Space Environ Med. 2007;78(4 Suppl):A56–66.

22. Kaiserman I, Hazarbassanov R, Varssano D, Grinbaum A. Contrast sensitivity after wave front-guided LASIK. Ophthalmology. 2004;111(3):454–7. doi:10.1016/j.ophtha.2003.06.017.

23. Kim JY, Kim MJ, Kim TI, Choi HJ, Pak JH, Tchah H. A femtosecond laser creates a stronger flap than a mechanical microkeratome. Invest Ophthalmol Vis Sci. 2006;47(2):599–604. doi:10.1167/iovs.05-0458.

24. Knorz MC, Vossmerbaeumer U. Comparison of flap adhesion strength using the Amadeus microkeratome and the IntraLase iFS femtosecond laser in rabbits. J Refract Surg. 2008; 24(9):875–8.

25. Laurent JM, Schallhorn SC, Spigelmire JR, Tanzer DJ. Stability of the laser in situ keratomileusis corneal flap in rabbit eyes. J Cataract Refract Surg. 2006;32(6):1046–51. doi:10.1016/j.jcrs.2006.02.038.

26. Lindstrom RL, Macrae SM, Pepose JS, Hoopes PC Sr. Corneal inlays for presbyopia correction. Curr Opin Ophthalmol. 2013;24(4):281–7. doi:10.1097/ICU.0b013e328362293e.

27. Mader TH, Blanton CL, Gilbert BN, Kubis KC, Schallhorn SC, White LJ, Parmley VC, Ng JD. Refractive changes during 72-hour exposure to high altitude after refractive surgery. Ophthalmology. 1996;103(8):1188–95. doi:10.1016/s0161-6420(96)30523-x.

28. Mader TH, Koch DD, Manuel K, Gibson CR, Effenhauser RK, Musgrave S. Stability of vision during space flight in an astronaut with bilateral intraocular lenses. Am J Ophthalmol. 1999;127(3):342–3.

29. Maguen E, Nesburn AB, Salz JJ. Bilateral photorefractive keratectomy with intentional unilateral undercorrection in an aircraft pilot. J Cataract Refract Surg. 1997;23(2):294–6.

30. McDonald MB, Durrie D, Asbell P, Maloney R, Nichamin L. Treatment of presbyopia with conductive keratoplasty: six-month results of the 1-year United States FDA clinical trial. Cornea. 2004;23(7):661–8.

31. McDonald MB, Hersh PS, Manche EE, Maloney RK, Davidorf J, Sabry M, Conductive Keratoplasty United States Investigators G. Conductive keratoplasty for the correction of low to moderate hyperopia: U.S. clinical trial 1-year results on 355 eyes. Ophthalmology. 2002;109(11):1978–89. discussion 1989–1990

32. Moon CH. Four-year visual outcomes after photorefractive keratectomy in pilots with low-moderate myopia. Br J Ophthalmol. 2016;100(2):253–7. doi:10.1136/bjophthalmol-2015-306967.

33. Munoz G, Albarran-Diego C, Sakla HF, Javaloy J, Alio JL. Transient light-sensitivity syndrome after laser in situ keratomileusis with the femtosecond laser Incidence and prevention. J Cataract Refract Surg. 2006;32(12):2075–9. doi:10.1016/j.jcrs.2006.07.024.

34. Nakagawara VB, Loochan FK, Wood KJ. Aphakia and artificial lens implants in the civil airman population. Aviat Space Environ Med. 1993;64(10):932–8.

35. Nakagawara VB, Montgomery RW, Wood KJ. Aviation accidents and incidents associated with the use of ophthalmic devices by civilian pilots. Aviat Space Environ Med. 2002; 73(11):1109–13.

36. Nakagawara VB, Veronneau SJ. Monovision contact lens use in the aviation environment: a report of a contact lens-related aircraft accident. Optometry. 2000;71(6):390–5.

37. Nakagawara VB, Wood KJ, Medicine USOoA, Civil Aeromedical Institute. The aeromedical certification of photorefractive keratectomy in civil aviation: a reference guide. Washington, D.C.: U.S. Department of Transportation, Federal Aviation Administration, Office of Aviation Medicine. (1998). https://www.faa.gov/data_research/research/med_humanfacs/oamtechreports/1990s/media/AM98-25.pdf.

38. Nakagawara VB, Wood KJ, Montgomery RW. Information for pilots considering laser eye surgery. Federal Aviation Administration. https://www.faa.gov/pilots/safety/pilotsafetybrochures/media/LaserEye_II.pdf. Accessed July 2016.

39. Nakagawara VB, Wood KJ, Montgomery RW. The use of contact lenses by US civilian pilots. Optometry. 2002;73(11):674–84.

40. National Research Council (US) Working Group on Contact Lens Use under Adverse Conditions. Contact lens use under adverse conditions: applications in military aviation. Washington, DC: National Academy Press; 1990.

41. O'Brart DP, Lohmann CP, Fitzke FW, Klonos G, Corbett MC, Kerr-Muir MG, Marshall J. Discrimination between the origins and functional implications of haze and halo at night after photorefractive keratectomy. J Refract Corneal Surg. 1994;10(2 Suppl):S281.

42. O'Connell SR, Markovits AS. The fate of eyewear in aircraft ejections. Aviat Space Environ Med. 1995;66(2):104–7.
43. Parson S. The eyes have it. FAA Safety Briefing. 2013;52(1):24–7. https://www.faa.gov/news/safety_briefing/2013/media/JanFeb2013.pdf.
44. Pietila J, Makinen P, Pajari T, Suominen S, Keski-Nisula J, Sipila K, Huhtala A, Uusitalo H. Eight-year follow-up of photorefractive keratectomy for myopia. J Refract Surg. 2004;20(2):110–5.
45. Rafnsson V, Olafsdottir E, Hrafnkelsson J, Sasaki H, Arnarsson A, Jonasson F. Cosmic radiation increases the risk of nuclear cataract in airline pilots: a population-based case-control study. Arch Ophthalmol. 2005;123(8):1102–5. doi:10.1001/archopht.123.8.1102.
46. Reinstein DZ, Archer TJ, Randleman JB. Mathematical model to compare the relative tensile strength of the cornea after PRK, LASIK, and small incision lenticule extraction. J Refract Surg. 2013;29(7):454–60. doi:10.3928/1081597X-20130617-03.
47. Rings M (2001) Ocular trauma in aviation: a review of navy mishaps 1980–2000. Paper presented at the Aerospace Medical Association 72nd Annual Scientific Meeting, Reno, 2001.
48. Schallhorn S, Tanzer D (2006) Advancing the science of wavefront guided ablation. Paper presented at the American Academy of Ophthalmology Annual Meeting, Las Vegas, 2006.
49. Schallhorn S, Tanzer D, Sanders DR, Sanders ML. Randomized prospective comparison of visian toric implantable collamer lens and conventional photorefractive keratectomy for moderate to high myopic astigmatism. J Refract Surg. 2007;23(9):853–67.
50. Schallhorn SC, Blanton CL, Kaupp SE, Sutphin J, Gordon M, Goforth H Jr, Butler FK Jr. Preliminary results of photorefractive keratectomy in active-duty United States Navy personnel. Ophthalmology. 1996;103(1):5–22.
51. Schallhorn SC, Tanzer DJ, Kaupp SE, Brown M, Malady SE. Comparison of night driving performance after wavefront-guided and conventional LASIK for moderate myopia. Ophthalmology. 2009;116(4):702–9. doi:10.1016/j.ophtha.2008.12.038.
52. Schallhorn SC, Venter JA, Hannan SJ, Hettinger KA. Wavefront-guided photorefractive keratectomy with the use of a new Hartmann-Shack aberrometer in patients with myopia and compound myopic astigmatism. J Ophthalmol. 2015;2015:514837. doi:10.1155/2015/514837.
53. Stanley PF, Tanzer DJ, Schallhorn SC. Laser refractive surgery in the United States Navy. Curr Opin Ophthalmol. 2008;19(4):321–4. doi:10.1097/ICU.0b013e3283009ee3.
54. Still D, Temme L. Eyeglass use by U.S. Navy jet pilots: effects on night carrier landing performance. Aviat Space Environ Med. 1992;63(4):273–5.
55. Tanna M, Schallhorn SC, Hettinger KA. Femtosecond laser versus mechanical microkeratome: a retrospective comparison of visual outcomes at 3 months. J Refract Surg. 2009;25(7 Suppl):S668–71.
56. Tanzer DJ, Brunstetter T, Zeber R, Hofmeister E, Kaupp S, Kelly N, Mirzaoff M, Sray W, Brown M, Schallhorn S. Laser in situ keratomileusis in United States Naval aviators. J Cataract Refract Surg. 2013;39(7):1047–58. doi:10.1016/j.jcrs.2013.01.046.
57. Tanzer DJ, Schallhorn S (2006) Comparison visual outcomes of mechanical and femtosecond keratomes in wavefront-guided LASIK. Paper presented at the American Academy of Ophthalmology Annual Meeting, Las Vegas, 2006.
58. Tanzer DJ, Schallhorn SC, Brown MC. Ejection from an aircraft following photorefractive keratectomy: a case report. Aviat Space Environ Med. 2000;71(10):1057–9.
59. Temme L, Still D. Prescriptive eyeglass use by U.S. Navy jet pilots: effects on air-to-air target detection. Aviat Space Environ Med. 1991;62(9 Pt 1):823–6.
60. Temme LA. Naval aviation vision standards research at the Naval Aerospace Medical Research Laboratory: the long view. Defense Technical Information Center. (1993). http://www.dtic.mil/dtic/tr/fulltext/u2/a275885.pdf.
61. Teus MA, de Benito-Llopis L, Alio JL. Mitomycin C in corneal refractive surgery. Surv Ophthalmol. 2009;54(4):487–502. doi:10.1016/j.survophthal.2009.04.002.
62. Van de Pol C, Greig JL, Estrada A, Bissette GM, Bower KS. Visual and flight performance recovery after PRK or LASIK in helicopter pilots. Aviat Space Environ Med. 2007;78(6):547–53.

63. Wiley RW. Military research with contact lenses. (1993). U.S. Army Aeromedical Research Laboratory. http://www.dtic.mil/dtic/tr/fulltext/u2/a267377.pdf.
64. Wright ST, Ivan DJ, Clark PJ, Gooch JM, Thompson W. Corrective lens use and refractive error among United States Air Force aircrew. Mil Med. 2010;175(3):197–201.
65. Zhang Y, Shen Q, Jia Y, Zhou D, Zhou J. Clinical outcomes of SMILE and FS-LASIK used to treat myopia: a meta-analysis. J Refract Surg. 2016;32(4):256–65. doi:10.3928/1081597X-20151111-06.
66. Richmond CJ, Barker PD, Levine EM, Hofmeister EM. Laser in situ keratomileusis flap stability in an aviator following aircraft ejection. J Cataract Refract Surg. 2016;42(11):1681–3.
67. FDA approves VisuMax Femtosecond Laser to surgically treat nearsightedness. US Food and Drug Administration. https://www.fda.gov/NewsEvents/Newsroom/PressAnnouncements/ucm520560.htm. Accessed 14 May 2017.

Chapter 4
Night Vision and Military Operations

Kraig S. Bower, Rose Kristine C. Sia, Denise S. Ryan, Bruce A. Rivers,
Tana Maurer, and Jeff Rabin

Night Vision

The human eye has the ability to see in a wide range of light intensity spanning
nearly ten log units. Visual processing, including spatial detection, discrimination
and recognition, temporal vision, color vision, as well as peripheral and night vision
are predicated on normal retinal function which includes both rod (low-light, nighttime) and cone (higher light, daytime) retinal photoreceptors. Importantly, these
duplex systems do not operate independently but interact to allow a continuum of
optimal vision performance. Under high light conditions (e.g., clear sunny day), the
photopic division of the visual system is utilized; cone photoreceptors are active
allowing high visual acuity and color perception. Under very low light conditions
(e.g., starlight), the visual system switches to scotopic division; rod photoreceptors
become primarily active mediating low light-sensitivity, with decreased visual acuity and color perception. Mesopic vision operates under intermediate illumination
(e.g. moonlight); rods and cones are both active allowing for enhanced sensitivity,
color vision and usable visual acuity [81] (Fig. 4.1). The eye usually adapts rapidly

The views expressed in this chapter are those of the authors and do not reflect the official policy of
the Department of the Army/Navy/Air Force, Department of Defense, or the U.S. Government.

K.S. Bower, MD (✉)
Johns Hopkins University, Wilmer Eye Institute, Lutherville, MD, USA
e-mail: kbower5@jhmi.edu

R.K.C. Sia, MD • D.S. Ryan, MS • B.A. Rivers, MD, LTC
Fort Belvoir Community Hospital, Warfighter Refractive Eye Surgery Program and Research
Center, Fort Belvoir, VA, USA

T. Maurer, BS, ChE, MS EE
US Army RDECOM CERDEC NVESD, Fort Belvoir, VA, USA

J. Rabin, OD, MS, PhD
University of the Incarnate Word, Rosenberg School of Optometry, San Antonio, TX, USA

© Springer International Publishing AG 2017   55
P.S. Subramanian (ed.), *Ophthalmology in Extreme Environments*,
Essentials in Ophthalmology, DOI 10.1007/978-3-319-57600-8_4

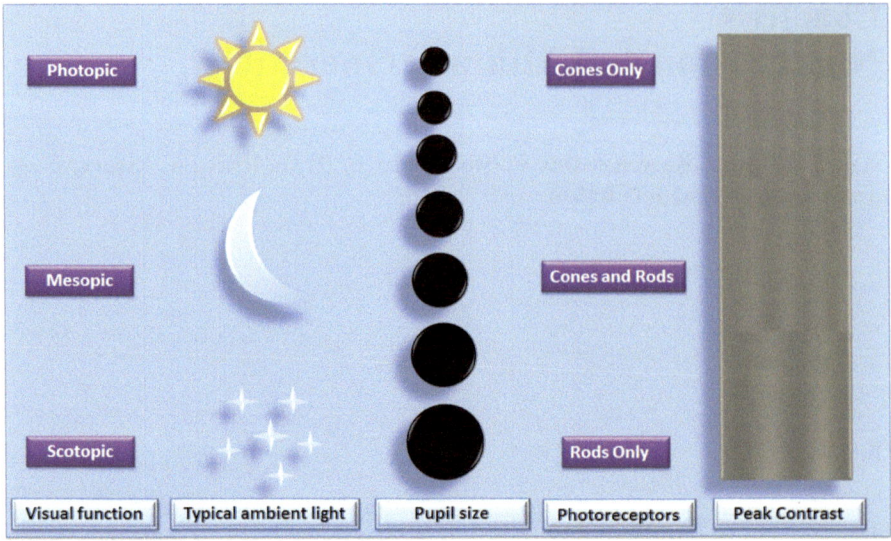

Fig. 4.1 Photopic, mesopic and scotopic visions. Photopic vision operates under high ambient light conditions (e.g. clear sunny day); mesopic vision functions under intermediate light conditions (e.g. moonlight) and scotopic vision operates under low light conditions (e.g. starlight). Pupil size varies according to ambient light levels, generally between 2 mm, in photopic level, and 8 mm, in scotopic level. Photopic vision is mediated by cone photoreceptors only, mesopic vision by both cones and rods and scotopic vision by rods only. Peak contrast sensitivity function is near 8 cycles per degree (cpd) at photopic level and decreases to near 1 cpd at scotopic level [74]

to changing background light levels. When shifting from photopic to scotopic conditions, recovery of light-sensitivity in the dark becomes slower following an exposure to bright light, a phenomenon called dark adaptation. In this process, the cone photoreceptors become completely dark-adapted first, occurring within 5–8 min (rapid phase) whereas rod photoreceptors take longer, about 40–50 min to fully adapt [52].

In the United States Military Physical Profile Serial System, visual acuity is used to evaluate an individual service member's physical visual capacity. As it is an assessment of the resolution limit of the visual system, it is a sensitive measure of changes in refractive error [78] and is conventionally used to assess overall visual function. The visual acuity standard is an essential component to determine enlistment induction, retention standards, military occupational specialty eligibility, and combat vision readiness [75]. Although screening for vision readiness may differ for each military service branch, visual acuity requirements remain nearly identical [22]. A minimum distance visual acuity of 20/40 in at least one eye with or without eyeglasses is required by the Army and Navy to determine vision readiness unless the occupational specialty calls for a more stringent requirement [22].

These standard visual acuity tests are an important baseline, but under certain circumstances they may not be sensitive enough to detect subtle visual changes. A study by Applegate and associates showed that in healthy individuals with excellent photopic high contrast visual acuities (i.e., 20/17 or better), variations in optical image quality did not appear to influence their performance when testing photopic high contrast visual acuity but it did impact their visual acuities under more challenging conditions, such as in low contrast and/or low luminance levels [2]. In another study by Subramanian and colleagues, a group of healthy volunteers from a Special Operations unit was tested for their best-corrected photopic visual acuity and their performance was observed to diminish with decreasing contrast level and night sky condition [64].Visual acuity, performed under mesopic and scotopic conditions, may be more sensitive to early visual functional changes which are valuable not only in detecting and monitoring ocular dysfunctions but also in predicting performance at night [5, 6].

In addition to visual acuity measurements, contrast sensitivity is also a significant measure of visual function in relation to perceived visual performance. As the 'real world' is composed of objects of varying sizes and contrasts, the clinical use of contrast sensitivity is based on the assumption that it can predict whether an individual has difficulty seeing objects encountered in everyday life [44]. In the military context, contrast sensitivity testing measures the ease or difficulty in detecting sizes and structural details of objects; given the variety of environments in which service members operate in, contrast sensitivity may be more operationally relevant than traditional letter chart acuity [66]. According to Barbur and Stockman [4], occupational environments usually contain stimuli three times the limit of spatial resolution. In military operational environments, target acquisition may require service members to perform at their resolution limits necessitating optimal resolution and contrast sensitivity to achieve optimal visual performance.

Night Vision Systems

Night vision involves different visual functions which may vary significantly with changing light levels. Changes in visual function are well-recognized and include decreased visual acuity in central and peripheral locations, as well as reduced contrast sensitivity for all spatial frequencies [77]. Night vision systems, such as image intensifiers and thermal imaging systems, have considerable capabilities and allow the expansion of night operations. Visualization through night vision systems has improved situational awareness and spatial orientation which in turn enhances navigation, threat detection, target acquisition and weapons deployment [32].

According to the Night Vision and Electronic Sensors Directorate, the development of image intensification systems began in the 1940s with the use of Sniperscopes during World War II (http://www.cerdec.army.mil/inside_cerdec/nvesd/history). While limited, Sniperscopes initiated more advanced night vision technology. The 1970s saw development of the first night vision goggles (NVGs) and use of forward looking infrared (FLIRs) systems for 'seeing' at night as well as through smoke, fog and other obscured conditions. Night vision systems progressed significantly in the subsequent years, expanding military capabilities, including aided target detection and recognition. Night vision technologies including NVG and FLIR have been crucial in recent conflicts, significantly enhancing operational capabilities and performance. Exploitation of night vision systems has significantly impacted night operations which is vital for around-the-clock combat readiness.

Under favorable ambient illumination such as a full moon and clear sky, the output luminance of NVGs is in the low photopic range whereas under more challenging ambient conditions such as overcast moonlight or starlight, the output luminance of an NVG is under mesopic range [12]. NVGs are designed to amplify ambient light (Fig. 4.2). Long wavelength visible and near infrared light (600–900 nm) are captured through an objective lens of the image intensification device and are sent to an infrared-sensitive photocathode which converts photons to electrons. The released electrons are then amplified within a microchannel plate. Once the electrons from the microchannel plate hit the phosphor screen, the electrons are converted back to photons creating a green visible image that can be viewed through an eyepiece (Fig. 4.3) [64]. Previous research has shown that NVG-aided visual acuity exceeds unaided visual acuity under the same ambient luminance conditions [39]. This, however does not imply that visual acuity will be as good as in the daytime. Under optimal night conditions, an individual with 20/20 daytime vision can expect no better than 20/50 vision with second-generation NVGs and 20/40 vision with third-generation NVGs [63, 70]. Furthermore, as NVG works by amplifying available light, NVG-aided visual acuity may be dependent on the display luminance of the NVG. This relationship may be mainly attributed to the quantal fluctuations in light intensity rather than optical factors such as accommodation, pupil size and/or high order aberrations [64]. The effectiveness of NVGs may be significantly reduced under conditions such as rain, snow, dust, haze, fog, and smoke [17].

Fig. 4.2 Sample imagery through an image intensification device

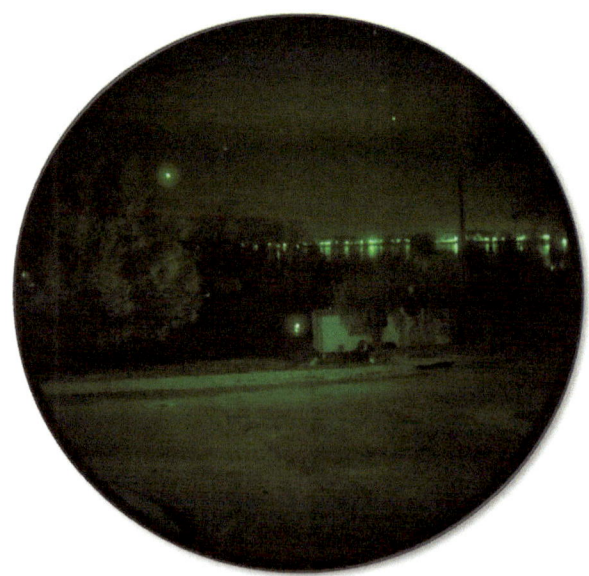

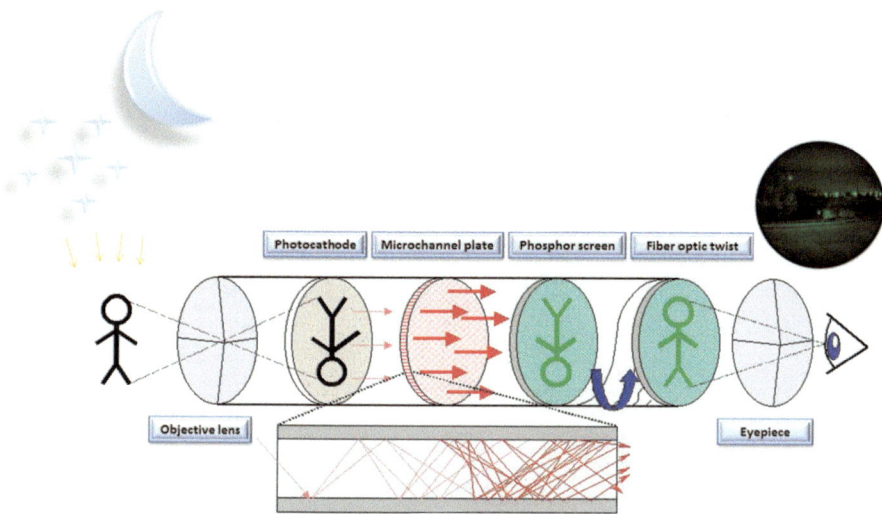

Fig. 4.3 Schematic representation of image intensification device i.e., night vision goggles (Adapted from Subramanian et al. [64])

Contrast sensitivity (CS), which assesses the ability to detect and/or recognize low contrast stationary or moving targets, can be decreased through NVGs. Both spatial and temporal contrast sensitivity were lower through NVGs compared to CS in response to stimuli presented without the NVGs in place but at brightness (luminance) and chromaticity (green color) levels which matched those of the NVG display. Hence CS can diminish through NVGs due to optical attenuation and electro-optical noise, even under optimal ambient levels of illumination [48, 49].

NVGs must be properly adjusted for optimal clarity and aligned to the visual axis to approach the best level of acuity. Aviators who are experienced in using NVGs have been shown to achieve visual acuity ranging from 20/50 to 20/55 with their 'usual' adjustment method. Visual acuity significantly improves to a range of 20/45 to 20/50 when adjustment is performed using the standard NVG resolution chart whereas visual acuity of 20/30 to 20/40 may be achieved with proper adjustment training such as in an NVG test lane [15]. Moreover, the prolonged use of improperly adjusted interpupillary distance on NVGs (e.g., PVS-5A) may induce shift in lateral phoria as a byproduct of additional convergent or divergent efforts. This has been implicated in reports of aviators failing stereoscopic depth perception tests after a prolonged flight training employing NVGs [61].

As part of the possible NVG adjustments, NVG systems have built-in spherical lens oculars allowing spherical refractive corrections ranging from +2.00 diopters of hyperopia to −6.00 diopters of myopia. Astigmatism of up to ±1.00 diopter may be corrected by spherical equivalent [19]. Prior to the availability of refractive surgery in the military, older models of NVGs such as AN/PVS-5 and 5A were incompatible with aviators with refractive error. These "full frame" goggles have an occluding face-plate (Fig. 4.4) which precluded the use of spectacles for individuals with refractive errors exceeding the corrective limits of the goggles [19].

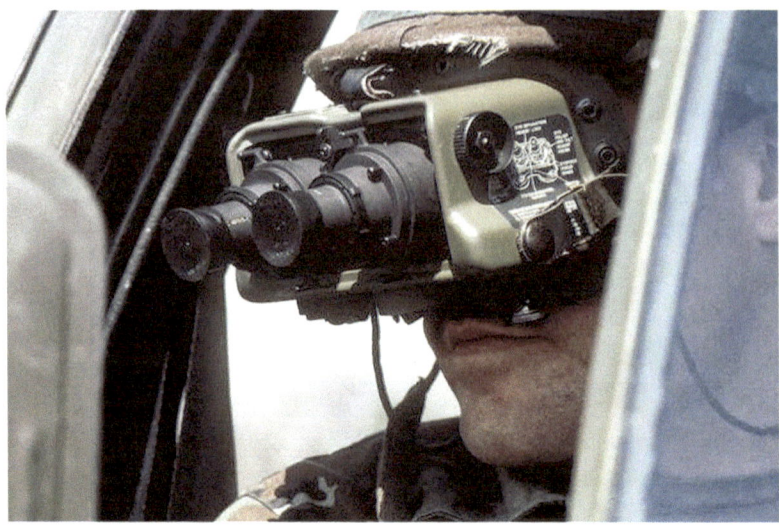

Fig. 4.4 AN/PVS-5 night vision "full frame" goggles

Another challenge presented to users of night vision systems is display luminance and the impediments associated with switching between two types of imaging devices from higher luminance to lower luminance. Luminance of the NVG
display is typically in the mesopic to low photopic range (0.3–2.0 foot-lambert) and
remains relatively constant in any one night sky condition whereas luminance of the
FLIR display can be adjusted to be nearly 100 times brighter than the NVG display
(Fig. 4.5). In a simulated experiment, the investigators demonstrated that shifting
from higher to lower luminance may increase adaptation demands causing transient
visual loss of up to 4 s, reduction of visual acuity and contrast sensitivity [50].
Recent developments in next generation devices which combine image intensification and forward looking infrared systems will attempt to highlight the benefits and
reduce the limitations of both systems.

Challenges in Night Vision

Night vision, whether aided or unaided, is susceptible to several physiologic factors.
It is known that certain ocular diseases such as retinitis pigmentosa as well as lack of
essential nutrients such as Vitamin A and zinc can decrease night vision. Moreover,
in healthy individuals various factors including age, pupil size, astigmatism [6, 46,
67] as well as oxygenation [11] and acceleration can impair visual performance at
night [68]. Dark adaptation gradually slows down and mesopic and scotopic visual
performance decline with age during adulthood [26, 27, 46]. Healthy older adults
require significantly more time to dark adapt compared to younger adults [27]. Pupil
size generally varies between 2 and 8 mm when shifting from bright light to very

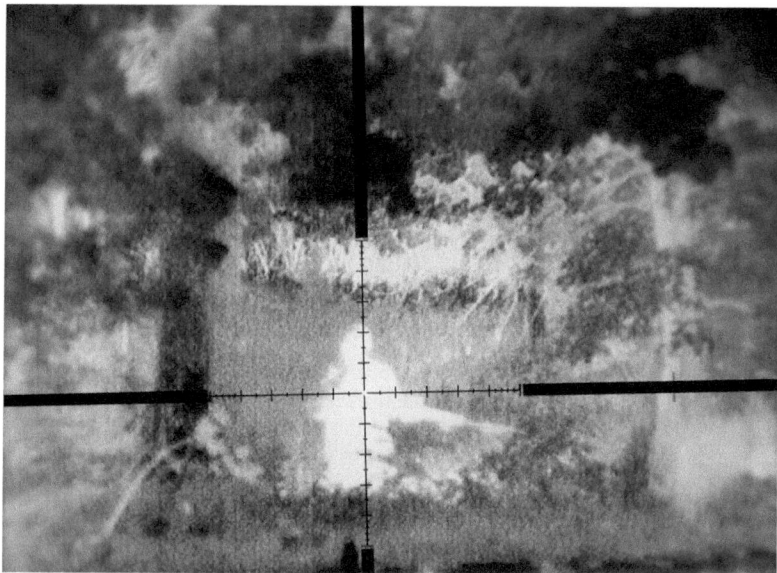

Fig. 4.5 Sample imagery through a forward looking infrared device

dark conditions. Under low light, increased pupil size reduces retinal image quality due to increased higher order aberrations, such as spherical aberration and coma, as well as light scatter in the eye which in turn, decreases visual acuity and contrast sensitivity [4]. Uncorrected astigmatism may lead to non-optimal NVG visual acuity. Astigmatism <1.00 diopter have minimal impact while greater amounts of uncorrected astigmatism significantly decrease NVG acuity [31]. Consistent with this finding, astigmatism exceeding 0.75 diopters may result in greater mesopic visual function complaints in post-refractive surgery patients [30].

Another challenge to vision is high altitude. Aviators as well as ground forces operating in a high altitude environment may be exposed to hypobaric hypoxic stress. A mild hypoxic state, like breathing air at an altitude of 10,000 ft (3048 m) for a short duration, can diminish visual performance progressively with decreasing light conditions. Furthermore, reduced mesopic visual acuity and contrast sensitivity may also be observed in an even milder hypoxic state (equivalent to breathing at 8000 ft or 2438 m). On the other hand, supplemental oxygen appears to improve low contrast acuity and can extend functionally useful vision to lower light levels suggesting that visual performance is oxygen-dependent [10, 11]. Continued impairment of night vision may be manifested during sustained hypoxic state such as during a sojourn at high altitude. The effects of high altitude to dark adaptation are rapid and sensitive. Hypoxia can have a critical and systematic degrading influence on the efficiency of dark adaptation. This effect was observed during a course of high altitude exposure which was more apparent during the first 10 min. Recovery also appeared to be rapid and substantial upon return to sea level or oxygen supplementation [33].

While NVGs are normally used when visual capabilities are unimpaired by oxygen deprivation, use of NVGs at high altitudes could potentially impair performance. However, NVG-aided contrast sensitivity appears relatively unaffected by oxygenation state. The preservation of the NVG-aided contrast sensitivity is possibly due to its dependency on the goggles' gain [12, 13, 72].

Visual changes are well-recognized consequences of exposure to high-speeds. With modern weaponry and vehicle performance, service members, such as fighter pilots, may also be subjected to high accelerations. In this environment, there is a significant rise in mesopic luminance threshold (i.e., reduced sensitivity) at +2 Gz, +3 Gz (head to foot acceleration) and +2 Gy (lateral acceleration). Reduced contrast sensitivity may be due to decreased retinal blood supply secondary to blood shifting to lower extremities, reduced cardiac output and/or cerebrovascular constriction associated with hyperventilation. Blood shift may be the primary factor contributing to the changes in contrast sensitivity in +2 Gz and +3 Gz environments but not in a + 2 Gy environment [68]. Specialized trainings such as anti-G straining maneuvers [20] have allowed military pilots as well as astronauts to increase tolerance to high acceleration and safely operate under such conditions.

Night Performance

Marksmanship is a common task for all military service members. For these individuals, effectively engaging a target undoubtedly calls for adequate visual performance. One study observed that individuals with visual acuity of 20/32 or better were more likely to hit a target [22]. Another study showed that the number of missed targets doubled at 20/50 resulting in 71% decrease of marksmanship performance [75]. Both studies indicate that marksmanship is affected by visual acuity at daytime and at nighttime [75] and corroborate the validity of the vision classification system and the importance of the aforementioned vision readiness standards of the U.S. military. These studies also highlighted the importance of vision correction to maximize vision performance, especially for deployed military.

Night driving entails mesopic vision as ambient light sources are usually available during operations. Under limited illumination, driving at night is considerably more visually demanding than driving during the day. Recognition of road signs, obstacles and pedestrians while driving at night can be significantly degraded under low light conditions, and this problem may be more pronounced in older drivers [77]. Overall nighttime driving performance is significantly impacted by reduced visual acuity compared to daytime conditions [76]. There is also a greater risk of nighttime accidents with reduced mesopic vision and increased glare sensitivity [3]. In the military, there are certain instances when service members are required to drive during periods of darkness and limited visibility. Such missions are carefully planned in order to avoid catastrophes as more accidents and incidents are encountered during night operations than their day-time counterparts [28]. Availability of image intensification systems offers wheeled vehicle operators the ability to accomplish their mission even in conditions that would not otherwise be possible. Military manuals are available to address techniques and procedures and specific considerations for using NVGs for driving. Driving using NVGs safely and effectively depends on the operator's overall proficiency in NVG use and habituation under these conditions, to include a limited field of view and ambient light adjustments.

The daily tasks of military service members include the ability to discriminate objects of military relevance. An object of interest may provide visual clues to help discriminate between friendly forces, combatants and civilian/non-combatants. The hierarchy of target acquisition begins with a target being detected as militarily rel-evant which may be followed by an action to perform higher levels of discrimina-tion, such as classification, recognition, and identification. Typical target acquisition tasks may include detection and identification of combat vehicles, detection of per-sonnel, and discrimination between handheld objects and weapons. The U.S. mili-tary rules of engagement generally require positive identification of a target prior to action, such as use of force against an enemy target [38].

Before the identification of a target can take place, one has to locate the target first. Locating a possible target occurs during a search task. Generally, a search task consists of an operator viewing a specific portion of a scene and, if an imag-ing system is used, the operator adjusts the device to get a better look at any "tar-get like" areas encountered to determine if a target is, in fact, present [38]. During scotopic search, studies have shown that scotopic contrast sensitivity is signifi-cantly reduced with a functional scotoma in the fovea. When the fovea is not functional, the brain adjusts to meet some properties of rod vision. This implies that humans are able to modify their search behavior as ambient light level decreases [45]. In a search and rescue exercise at sea, visual acuity and color vision did not seem to correlate with life raft detection using NVGs, which seems reasonable since NVGs use only a single green color to identify objects and life raft detection likely involves detection of low spatial frequencies which are less acuity dependent. The combination of life raft light and NVGs in night searches seemed to be as effective as daytime searches with unlit rafts. Night searches for unlit rafts were influenced by weather conditions and not by individual differ-ences. As NVGs amplified life raft light, detectability was not limited by human performance and weather conditions [16]. Once a target has been detected and localized, it can be identified. The ability to identify military targets at night has been shown to directly correlate with dark adaptation, scotopic retinal sensitivity and contrast sensitivity under mesopic condition but not visual acuity. However, only scotopic retinal sensitivity and mesopic contrast sensitivity metrics are reproducible, making them suitable for assessing night vision ability in pilots and military personnel [35].

Refractive Surgery

Military personnel rely on visual performance and a reliable way to improve this performance is to enhance the warfighter's vision with refractive procedures that reduce or eliminate dependence on corrective lenses. There are several benefits that refractive surgery offers over glasses or optical inserts in a military context. It optimizes vision without the constraints of glasses, which may break, get scratched, or degrade due to environmental conditions (fog, rain, salt spray, sand etc.). Optical inserts which correct vision in masks can become dislodged or may limit peripheral vision. Sophisticated weapon systems can require goggles, headgear, or ballistic protection whose functionality may be impeded by glasses.

Contact lens wear can eliminate some of the interface obstacles inherent with spectacles, but aside from exceptions for authorized Air Force Personnel, use during deployment is prohibited by Department of Defense policy. This prohibition is a consequence of numerous cases of contact-lens related issues including keratitis, ulcers and infiltrates (DOD policy, [14, 69]). Refractive procedures avoid these aforementioned shortcomings. In fact, given operational demands and environmental extremes, there is no other profession that has benefited as greatly from refractive surgery as the military [7, 21, 58, 64, 65, 71].

Not only is refractive surgery an operational amplifier, refractive surgery enhances the quality of life and individual readiness of service members. A survey of Naval Aviators who underwent LASIK showed 95.9% of aviators felt improvement in their individual readiness and overwhelmingly would recommend the surgery to others (99.6%) [65]. These findings were similar to a review of the Army's Warfighter Refractive Eye Surgery Program (WRESP) of Soldiers returning from deployment [55]. Respondents were asked to rate how their capabilities changed in relation to the following tasks as a result of their refractive surgery: weapon sighting ability, night operations, ability to weather extreme environmental conditions, and use of personal protective equipment. Their capabilities in accomplishing the following tasks were rated as "better" or "much better" in weapon sighting ability (91.4%), use of night vision goggles (86.2%), operations in extreme environments (74.2%) and use of personal protective equipment (88%). When asked to rate the impact of refractive surgery on their deployment, 95.2% of soldiers felt their individual readiness was "better" or "much better", while 93.4% felt they were better able to contribute to their unit's mission [21, 55]. Refractive surgery also provides an opportunity for Service members to apply for occupational specialties for which they were previously not eligible due to restrictions of uncorrected visual acuity or refractive error, augmenting the pool of applicants to specialty programs, such as Aviation and Special Forces [21, 65].

While refractive surgery reduces the dependence on glasses, studies on vision after treatment with conventional lasers have reported reduced contrast sensitivity [8, 9, 25, 57]. The reduction of contrast sensitivity has been attributed to an observed multifactorial increase in higher order aberrations (HOA) [36, 43, 47, 79]. The lower order aberrations are typically referred to as the refraction of the eye in the form of sphere, cylinder and axis. HOAs such as coma, spherical aberration, and trefoil, especially when aggregated, can negatively influence visual performance [36]. The relationship between vision performance and HOAs is complicated and improvements in laser technology have reduced but not eliminated the adverse effects of the refractive-surgery induced HOAs [23, 34, 37, 40, 60, 62, 65, 73, 80, 82].

Even though studies have reported a correlation between contrast sensitivity function and performance tasks [42, 44], the change in contrast sensitivity after refractive surgery has not been found to correlate with task performance [38, 56, 66]. Although measurable under clinical conditions after refractive surgery, reduced contrast sensitivity is difficult to directly correlate with decreased functional performance [60, 71]. Observing changes in functional performance may be challenging to parse out due to the multifaceted involvement of senses, complexity of the task, and adaptation to visual changes post refractive surgery. Furthermore, [71] suggested experience may overcome visual decrements in controlled flight tasks. However, a study by Kaupp and associates did find a correlation between clinical measures of quality of vision and night driving visual performance [29]. Ongoing performance studies are underway at Warfighter Refractive Eye Surgery Programs to continue to explore this interaction and to continue low contrast, low light and vision analysis.

The advent of advanced lasers has, in addition to diminishing the reduction in contrast sensitivity, reduced night vision difficulties such as increased sensitivity to glare and appearance of halos after refractive surgery [34, 37, 41, 60, 65, 73, 82]. As reported by Maurer et al. [38], night vision symptoms increase in conditions where the pupil diameter is greatest (mesopic and scotopic) as a product of surgically-induced HOAs [38] Numerous studies have evaluated the performance profile of upgraded lasers, to include advanced laser ablation profiles, laser centration, and eye tracking, and have found improved outcomes and the moderation of some, but not all, of these symptoms [23, 60, 62] Furthermore, a study of contrast sensitivity after advanced laser ablation with either PRK or LASIK showed improvement from pre-operative performance (Fig. 4.6) [53]. While night vision disturbances secondary to large pupil size have been mitigated by both larger treatment zones and dynamic treatment profiles, it comes at the cost of increased tissue removal and possibly a more aggressive healing response. Multiple factors cause night vision problems and studies are ongoing to identify and quantify these factors. Ultimately, appropriate patient selection is still the most critical aspect of warfighter vision enhancement. Counseling of physical limitations (i.e. large pupil size, level of correction), age, realistic expectations, risks, technology available, and occupational limitations must all be considered when selecting appropriate candidates for refractive surgery.

There are some options to counter or neutralize night vision disturbances after refractive surgery. Additional wavefront-guided treatment after conventional surgery has been shown to moderate significant night vision symptoms [1, 51]. Pharmacological treatment has also been shown to transiently improve contrast sensitivity in patients with significant night vision symptoms post-refractive surgery [18]. Adoption of precision tools that have been developed, such as the enhanced night vision goggle (Fig. 4.7), a hybrid of image intensification and passive thermal

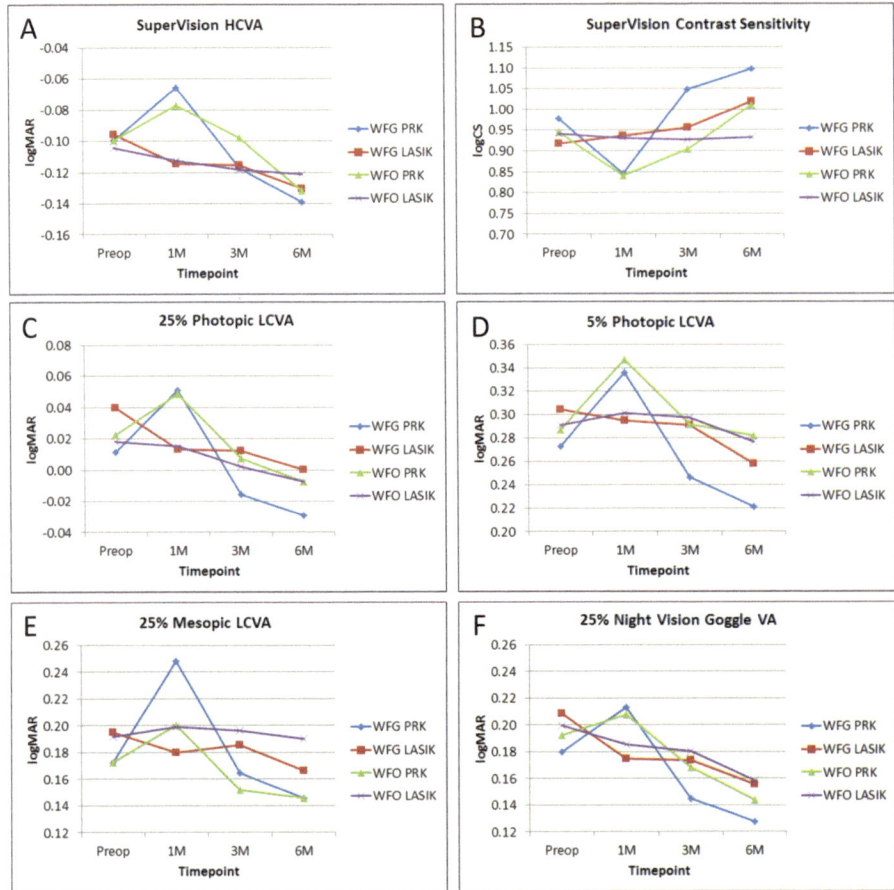

Fig. 4.6 Visual performance on SuperVision high contrast visual acuity (**a**) and contrast sensitivity (**b**); low-contrast visual acuity (LCVA): photopic visual acuity at 25 % contrast (**c**) and 5 % contrast (**d**); mesopic visual acuity at 25% contrast (**e**) and simulated night vision goggle (**f**) after wavefront-guided (WFG) PRK, wavefront-guided LASIK, wavefront-optimized (WFO) PRK and wavefront-optimized LASIK. For logMAR, decreased values indicate improvement. For logCS, increased values indicate improvement [53]

imaging, as well as thermal weapon sight, heightens visibility in inclement environments. However, these advanced tools must take into consideration the aforementioned challenges that may present when using image intensification devices: decreased sensitivity due to illumination conversely balanced with low light in which pupils dilate, increasing aberrations and scattered light.

A series of task performance studies have been completed to ascertain the impact of refractive surgery on night vision. Night firing studies using NVGs or a weapon-mounted forward-looking infrared (FLIR) thermal sight have shown uncorrected vision firing performance significantly improved postoperatively after photorefractive keratectomy (PRK) [7, 56, 64] and LASIK ([7], Ryan, unpublished

Fig. 4.7 Sample imagery
through Enhanced Night
Vision Goggles

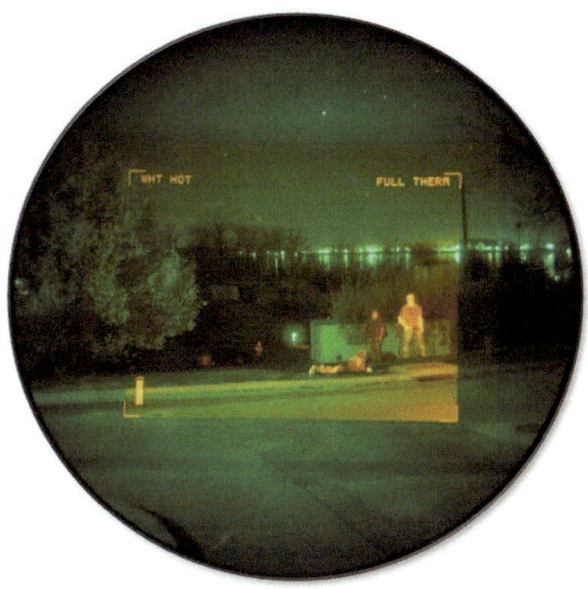

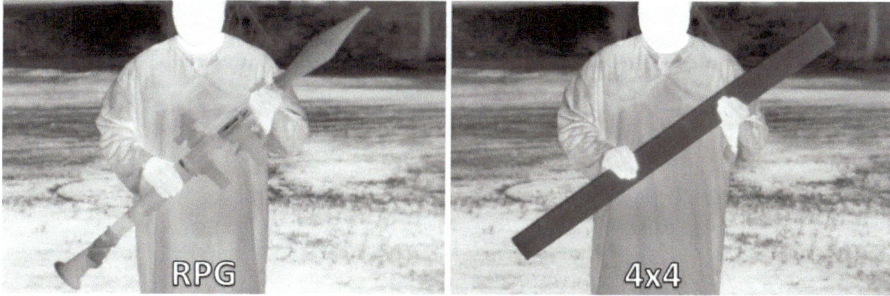

Fig. 4.8 Sample imagery from a computer-based handheld object identification training

data). Separate computer-based simulations (military target acquisition and driving) found an improvement in performance after advanced refractive surgery (Fig. 4.8) [38, 60]. Helicopter flight performance under day, night, unaided and NVG conditions found flight performance was unaffected after LASIK and PRK, notwithstanding a decrease in contrast visual performance [71]. Additional aviation considerations are discussed in the Chapter "Refractive Surgery in Aviators". While these studies support refractive enhancement of the warfighter, ongoing study of militarily relevant performance tasks is important to optimize patient selection and critically select appropriate innovative technology.

Compliance with Ethical Requirements

Conflict of Interest Kraig S. Bower, Rose K. Sia, Denise S. Ryan, Bruce A. Rivers, Tana Maurer, and Jeff C. Rabin declare that they have no conflict of interest.

Informed Consent No human studies were carried out by the authors for this article. No animal studies were carried out by the authors for this article.

References

1. Alio JL, Pinero D, Muftuoglu O. Corneal Wavefront-guided retreatments for significant night vision symptoms after myopic laser refractive surgery. Am J Ophthalmol. 2008;145:65–74.
2. Applegate RA, Marsack JD, Thibos LN. Metrics of retinal image quality predict visual performance in eyes with 20/17 or better visual acuity. Optom Vis Sci. 2006;83(9):635–40.
3. Babizhayev MA. Glare disability and driving safety. Ophthalmic Res. 2003;35(1):19–25.
4. Barbur JL, Stockman A. Photopic, mesopic and scotopic vision and changes in visual performance. In: Dartt DA, editor. Encyclopedia of the eye, vol. 3. Oxford: Academic; 2010. p. 323–31.
5. Barrio A, Antona B, Puell MC. Repeatability of mesopic visual acuity measurements using high- and low-contrast ETDRS letter charts. Graefes Arch Clin Exp Ophthalmol. 2015;253(5):791–5. doi:10.1007/s00417-014-2876-z. Epub 2014 Dec 9
6. Bartholomew AJ, Lad EM, Cao D, Bach M, Cirulli ET. Individual differences in scotopic visual acuity and contrast sensitivity: genetic and non-genetic influences. PLoS One. 2016;11(2):e0148192. doi:10.1371/journal.pone.0148192.
7. Bower KS, Burka JM, Subramanian PS, Stutzman RD, Mines MJ, Rabin JC. Night firing range performance following photorefractive keratectomy and laser in situ keratomileusis. Mil Med. 2006;171(6):468–71.
8. Chalita MR, Chavala S, Xu M, Krueger RR. Wavefront analysis in post-LASIK eyes and its correlation with visual symptoms, refraction, and topography. Ophthalmology. 2004;111:447–53.
9. Sharma M, Wachler BS, Chan CC. Higher order aberrations and relative risk of symptoms after LASIK. J Refract Surg. 2007;23:252–6.
10. Connolly DM. Oxygenation state and twilight vision at 2438 m. Aviat Space Environ Med. 2011;82(1):2–8.
11. Connolly DM, Barbur JL. Low contrast acuity at photopic and mesopic luminance under mild hypoxia, normoxia, and hyperoxia. Aviat Space Environ Med. 2009;80(11):933–40.
12. Connolly DM, Serle WP. Assisted night vision and oxygenation state: 'steady adapted gaze'. Aviat Space Environ Med. 2014;85(2):120–9.
13. Davis HQ, Kamimori GH, Kulesh DA, Mehm WJ, Anderson LH, Elsayed AM, Burge JR, Balkin TJ. Visual performance with the aviator night vision imaging system (ANVIS) at a simulated altitude of 4300 meters. Aviat Space Environ Med. 1995;66(5):430–4.
14. Department of the Army DA Pamphlet 40-506. The Army vision conservation and readiness program. 2009. http://armypubs.army.mil/epubs/pdf/p40_506.pdf. Accessed 20 June 2016.
15. DeVilbiss CA, Antonio JC. Measurement of night vision goggle (NVG) visual acuity with the NVG resolution chart. Aviat Space Environ Med. 1994;65(9):846–50.
16. Donderi DC. Visual acuity, color vision, and visual search performance at sea. Hum Factors. 1994;36(1):129–44.
17. Dyer JL, Young KM. Night vision goggle research and training issues for ground forces: a literature review. Army Research Inst for Behavioral and Social Sciences Fort Benning GA; 1998 May. No. ARI-TR-1082. http://www.dtic.mil/dtic/tr/fulltext/u2/a347071.pdf. Accessed: 20 June 2016.
18. Edwards JD, Burka JM, Bower KS, Stutzman RD, Sediq DA, Rabin JC. Effect of Brimonidine tartrate 0.15% on night-vision difficulty and contrast testing after refractive surgery. J Cataract Refract Surg. 2008;34:1538–41.

19. Farr WD. Compatibility of the aviation night vision imaging systems and the aging aviator. Aviat Space Environ Med. 1989;60(10 Pt 2):B78–80.
20. Gillingham KK, Fosdick JP. High-G training for fighter aircrew. Aviat Space Environ Med. 1998;59(1):12–9.
21. Hammond MD, Madigan WP, Bower KS. Refractive surgery in the United States Army, 2000–2003. Ophthalmology. 2005;112:184–90.
22. Hatch BC, Hilber DJ, Elledge JB, Stout JW, Lee RB. The effects of visual acuity on target discrimination and shooting performance. Optom Vis Sci. 2009;86(12):E1359–67. doi:10.1097/OPX.0b013e3181be9740.
23. He L, Manche LL. Prospective randomized contralateral eye evaluation of subjective quality of vision after wavefront-guided or wavefront-optimized photorefractive keratectomy. J Refract Surg. 2014;30(1):6–12.
24. U.S. Army Communications-Electronics Research, Development and Engineering Center. History of army night vision. 2015. http://www.cerdec.army.mil/inside_cerdec/nvesd/history. Accessed: 20 June 2016
25. Holladay JT, Dudeja DR, Chang J. Functional vision and corneal changes after laser in situ keratomileusis determined by contrast sensitivity, glare testing and corneal topography. J Cataract Refract Surg. 1999;25:663–9.
26. Jackson GR, Owsley C. Scotopic sensitivity during adulthood. Vis Res. 2000;40(18):2467–73.
27. Jackson GR, Owsley C, McGwin G Jr. Aging and dark adaptation. Vis Res. 1999;39(23):3975–82.
28. Johnson CW. The role of night vision equipment in military incidents and accidents. In: Johnson CW, Palanque P, editors. Human error, safety and systems development. IFIP International Federation for Information Processing, Vol. 152. Boston: Springer; 2004. p. 1–16.
29. Kaupp SE, Schallhorn SC, Tanzer DJ, Kelly NG, Malady SE, Brunstetter TJ. Prospective comparison of simulated night driving performance after wavefront guided treatments, both PRK and LASIK, for moderate and high myopia. Poster presented at the Association for Research in Vision and Ophthalmology annual meeting, Fort Lauderdale, May 2007.
30. Kezirian GM, Stonecipher KG. Subjective assessment of mesopic visual function after laser in situ keratomileusis. Ophthalmol Clin N Am. 2004 ;17(2):211–24, vii.
31. Kim HJ. Prevalence of astigmatism among aviators and its limiting effect upon visual performance with the AN/PVS-5 night vision goggles. 1982. http://www.dtic.mil/cgi-bin/GetTRDoc?Location=U2&doc=GetTRDoc.pdf&AD=ADA112836. Accessed 20 June 2016.
32. Knight KK, Apsey DA, Jackson WG, Dennis RJ. A comparison of stereopsis with ANVIS and F4949 night vision goggles. Aviat Space Environ Med. 1998;69(2):99–103.
33. Kobrick JL, Zwick H, Witt CE, Devine JA. Effects of extended hypoxia on night vision. Aviat Space Environ Med. 1984;55(3):191–5.
34. Lee HK, Choe CM, Ma KT, Kim EK. Measurement of contrast sensitivity and glare under mesopic and photopic conditions following wavefront-guided and conventional LASIK surgery. J Refract Surg. 2006;22(7):647–55.
35. Levy Y, Glovinsky Y. Evaluation of mid-term stability of night vision tests. Aviat Space Environ Med. 1997;68(7):565–8.
36. Lombardo M, Lombardo G. Wave aberration of human eyes and new descriptors of image optical quality and visual performance. J Cataract Refract Surg. 2010;36(2):313–31.
37. Mastropasqua L, Nubile M, Ciancaglini M, Toto L, Ballone E. Prospective randomized comparison of wavefront-guided and conventional photorefractive keratectomy for myopia with the meditec MEL 70 laser. J Refract Surg. 2004;20(5):422–31.
38. Maurer T, Deaver D, Howell C, Moyer S, Nguyen O, Mueller G, Ryan DS, Sia RK, Stutzman RD, Pasternak JF, Bower KS. Military target task performance after wavefront-guided (WFG) and wavefront-optimized (WFO) photorefractive keratectomy (PRK) Proc. SPIE. 9112, Sensing Technologies for Global Health, Military Medicine, and Environmental Monitoring IV, 91120U; 2014.
39. Monaco WA, Weatherless RA, Kalb JT. Enhancement of visual target detection with night vision goggles. 2006. http://www.dtic.mil/cgi-bin/GetTRDoc?AD=ADA448466. Accessed 20 June 2016.
40. Mrochen M, Donitzky C, Wüllner C, Löffler J. Wavefront-optimized ablation profiles: theoretical background. J Cataract Refract Surg. 2004;30:775–85.

41. Neeracher B, Senn P, Schipper I. Glare sensitivity and optical side effects 1 year after photorefractive keratectomy and laser in situ keratomileusis. J Cataract Refract Surg. 2004;30:1696–701.
42. O'Neal MR, Miller II, Robert E. Further investigation of contrast sensitivity and visual acuity in pilot detection of aircraft Wright-Patterson AFB, OH: Harry G Armstrong Aerospace Medical Research Lab. No. AAMRL-TR-88-002. 1998. http://www.dtic.mil/cgi-bin/GetTRD oc?Location=U2&doc=GetTRDoc.pdf&AD=ADA198434. Accessed 20 June 2016.
43. Oshika T, Okamoto C, Samejima T, Tokunaga T, Miyata K. Contrast sensitivity function and ocular higher-order wavefront aberrations in normal human eyes. Ophthalmology. 2006;113:1807–12.
44. Owsley C, Sloane ME. Contrast sensitivity, acuity, and the perception of 'real-world' targets. Br J Ophthalmol. 1987;71(10):791–6.
45. Paulun VC, Schütz AC, Michel MM, Geisler WS, Gegenfurtner KR. Visual search under scotopic lighting conditions. Vis Res. 2015;113(Pt B):155–68. doi:10.1016/j.visres.2015.05.004. Epub 2015 May 16
46. Puell MC, Palomo C, Sánchez-Ramos C, Villena C. Normal values for photopic and mesopic letter contrast sensitivity. J Refract Surg. 2004;20(5):484–8.
47. Quesnel NM, Lovasik JV, Ferremi C, Boileau M, Ieraci C. Laser in situ keratomileusis for myopia and the contrast sensitivity function. J Cataract Refract Surg. 2004;30(6):1209–18.
48. Rabin J. Spatial contrast sensitivity through aviator's night vision imaging system. Aviat Space Environ Med. 1993;64(8):706–10.
49. Rabin J, McLean W. A comparison between phosphors for aviators's night visión imaging system. Aviat Space Environ Med. 1996;67(5):429–33.
50. Rabin J, Wiley R. Switching from forward-looking infrared to night vision goggles: transitory effects on visual resolution. Aviat Space Environ Med. 1994;65(4):327–9.
51. Reinstein DZ, Archer TJ, Couch D, Schroeder E, Wotteke M. A new night vision disturbances parameter and contrast sensitivity as indicators of success in wavefront-guided enhancement. J Refract Surg. 2005;21:S535–40. doi:10.3928/1081-597X-20050901-23.
52. Reuter T. Fifty years of dark adaptation 1961–2011. Vis Res. 2011;51(21–22):2243–62. doi:10.1016/j.visres.2011.08.021. Epub 2011 Sep 6
53. Rivers BA, Ryan DS, Sia RK, Peppers L, Logan LA, Eaddy JB, Pasternak JF, Stutzman RD, Rodgers SB, Bower KS. Visual performance after wavefront-guided and wavefront-optimized Photorefractive Keratectomy (PRK) and Laser in situ keratomileusis (LASIK) Poster presented at the Association for Research in Vision and Ophthalmology annual meeting, Orlando, May 2014.
54. Rivers BA, Sia RK, Peppers L, Ryan DS, Rodgers SB. Validation of a military performance questionnaire for U.S. military service members with refractive error having refractive surgery. Poster presented at the American Society of Cataract and Refractive Surgery Annual Meeting. New Orleans, May 2016.
55. Ryan DS, Peppers L, Sia RK, Stutzman RD, Mines MJ, Wroblewski KJ, Bower KS. US soldiers' self-assessment of deployment after refractive surgery. Poster presented at the American Society of Cataract and Refractive Surgery Annual Meeting, Chicago, April 2012.
56. Ryan DS, Sia RK, Stutzman RD, Pasternak JF, Howard RS, Howell CL, Maurer T, Torres MF, Bower KS. Wavefront-guided versus wavefront-optimized photorefractive keratectomy: visual and military task performance. Military Med. 1636;182(1/2):2017.
57. Sakata N, Tokundaga T, Miyata K, Oshika T. Changes in contrast sensitivity function and ocular higher order aberration by conventional myopic photorefractive keratectomy. Jpn J Ophthalmol. 2007;51(5):347–52.
58. Schallhorn SC, Blanton CL, Kaupp SE, Sutphin J, Gordon M, Goforth H Jr, Butler FK Jr. Preliminary results of photorefractive keratectomy in active-duty US Navy personnel. Ophthalmology. 1996;103(1):5–22.
59. Schallhorn SC, Kaupp SE, Tanzer DJ, Tidwell J, Laurent J, Bourque LB. Pupil size and quality of vision after LASIK. Ophthalmology. 2003;110(8):1606–14
60. Schallhorn SC, Tanzer DJ, Kaupp SE, Brown M, Malady SE. Comparison of night driving performance after wavefront-guided and conventional LASIK for moderate myopia. Ophthalmology. 2009;116(4):702–9.

61. Sheehy JB, Wilkinson M. Depth perception after prolonged usage of night vision goggles. Aviat Space Environ Med. 1989;60(6):573–9.
62. Sia RK, Ryan DS, Stutzman RD, Pasternak JF, Eaddy JB, Logan LA, Torres MF, Bower KS. Wavefront-guided versus wavefront-optimized photorefractive keratectomy: clinical outcomes and patient satisfaction. J Cataract Refract Surg. 2015;41(10):2152–64.
63. Silberman WS, Apsey D, Ivan DJ, Jackson WG, Mitchell GW. The effect of test chart design and human factors on visual performance with night vision goggles. Aviat Space Environ Med. 1994;65(12):1077–81.
64. Subramanian PS, O'Kane B, Stefanik R, Stevens J, Rabin J, Bauer RM, Bower KS. Visual acuity and night vision performance after photorefractive keratectomy for myopia. Ophthalmology. 2003;110(3):525–30.
65. Tanzer DJ, Brunstetter T, Zeber R, Hofmeister E, Kaupp S, Kelly N, Mirazaoff M, Sray W, Brown M, Schallhorn S. Laser in situ keratomileusis in United States naval aviators. J Cataract Refract Surg. 2013;39(7):1047–58.
66. Temme LA, Ricks E, Morris A, Sherry D. Visual contrast sensitivity of U.S. Navy jet pilots. Aviat Space Environ Med. 1991;62(11):1032–6.
67. Thordsen JE, Bower KS, Warren BB, Stutzman R. Miotic effect of brimonidine tartrate 0.15% ophthalmic solution in normal eyes. J Cataract Refract Surg. 2004;30(8):1702–6.
68. Tipton DA, Marko AR, Ratino DA. The effects of acceleration forces on night vision. Aviat Space Environ Med. 1984;55(3):186–90.
69. USCENTCOM 021922Z DEC 11 Mod eleven to USCENTCOM. Individual protection and individual-unit deployment policy. 2011. http://www.cpms.osd.mil/expeditionary/pdf/MOD11-USCENTCOM-Indiv-Protection-Indiv-Unit-Deployment-Policy-Incl-Tab-A-and-B.pdf. Accessed 20 June 2016.
70. U.S. Army. Field Manual No. 3–22.9 Rifle marksmanship m16–/m4-series weapons. http://armypubs.army.mil/doctrine/DR_pubs/dr_a/pdf/fm3_22x9.pdf. Accessed 20 June 2016.
71. Van de Pol C, Greig JL, Estrada A, Bissette GM, Bower KS. Visual and flight performance recovery after PRK or LASIK in helicopter pilots. Aviat Space Environ Med. 2007;78(6):547–53.
72. Vecchi D, Morgagni F, Guadagno AG, Lucertini M. Visual function at altitude under night vision assisted conditions. Aviat Space Environ Med. 2014;85(1):60–5.
73. Villarrubia A, Palacín E, Bains R, Gersol J. Comparison of custom ablation and conventional laser in situ keratomileusis for myopia and myopic astigmatism using the Alcon excimer laser. Cornea. 2009;28(9):971–5.
74. Wandell BA. Pattern sensitivity. Foundations of vision. 1995. https://foundationsofvision.stanford.edu/chapter-7-pattern-sensitivity. Accessed 2 Jul 2016.
75. Wells KH, Wagner H, Reich LN, Hardigan PC. Military readiness: an exploration of the relationship between marksmanship and visual acuity. Mil Med. 2009;174(4):398–402.
76. Wood JM, Collins MJ, Chaparro A, Marszalek A, Carberry T, Lacherez P, Chu BS. Differential effects of refractive blur on day and nighttime driving performance. Invest Ophthalmol Vis Sci. 2014;55(4):2284–9. doi:10.1167/iovs.13-13369.
77. Wood JM, Owens DA. Standard measures of visual acuity do not predict drivers' recognition performance under day or night conditions. Optom Vis Sci. 2005;2(8):698–705.
78. Woods RL, Wood JM. The role of contrast sensitivity charts and contrast letter charts in clinical practice. Clin Exp Optom. 1995;78(2):42–57.
79. Yamane N, Miyata K, Samejima T, Hiraoka T, Kiuchi T, Okamoto F, Hirohara Y, Mihashi T, Oshika T. Ocular higher-order aberrations and contrast sensitivity after conventional laser in situ keratomileusis. Invest Ophthalmol Vis Sci. 2004;45(11):3986–90.
80. Yu J, Chen H, Wang F. Patient satisfaction and visual symptoms after wavefront-guided and wavefront-optimized LASIK with the WaveLight platform. J Refract Surg. 2008;24:477–86.
81. Zele AJ, Cao D. Vision under mesopic and scotopic illumination. Front Psychol. 2015;5:1594. doi:10.3389/fpsyg.2014.01594.
82. Zhang J, Zhou YH, Li R, Tian L. Visual performance after conventional LASIK and wavefront-guided LASIK with iris-registration: results at 1 year. Int J Ophthalmol. 2013;6(4):498–504.

Chapter 5
Deep-Sea Environments and the Eye

John Berdahl and Michael Greenwood

Introduction

The eye and body are exposed to a constant ambient pressure that comes from the weight of all of the gases in the earth's atmosphere. This pressure is not perceived by most people because it is a constant part of the environment and thus not part of conscious sensory attention. At sea level this pressure is approximately 760 mmHg, which is defined as 1 atmosphere (atm) of pressure. Entering a deep-sea environment exposes the eye to increased ambient pressures that involve a new set of potential ocular disorders. It also raises questions in regard to what is safe for patients. In this chapter, we will discuss how exposure to deep-sea environments can affect the eye.

Basic Principles

A review of some basic terminology and laws of physics is helpful in the understanding of how the eye is affected in the deep-sea environment. As stated above, at sea level the body (and the eye) is exposed to 760 mmHg, which is equivalent to 1 atm or 33 ft of seawater (FSW). These pressures are often used as a reference point from which other pressures are measured, which is also known as a gauge pressure. This is true for measurements performed via Goldmann applanation tonometry (GAT). Although often referred to as the intraocular pressure (IOP), this is a measurement of the difference between the inside of the eye and the external

J. Berdahl, MD (✉) • M. Greenwood, MD
Vance Thompson Vision, Sioux Falls, SD, USA
e-mail: johnberdahl@gmail.com

© Springer International Publishing AG 2017
P.S. Subramanian (ed.), *Ophthalmology in Extreme Environments*,
Essentials in Ophthalmology, DOI 10.1007/978-3-319-57600-8_5

Fig. 5.1 Normal
atmospheric and
intraocular pressures at sea
level. Note that the
transcorneal pressure
difference is 15

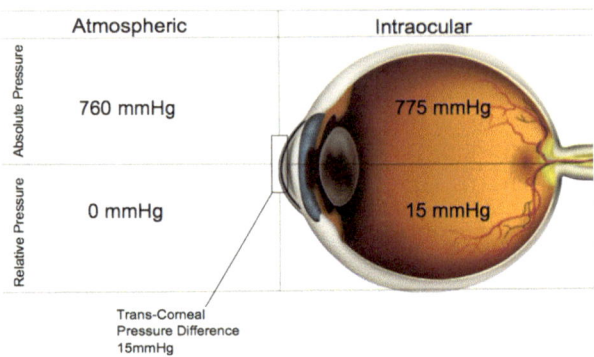

Normal Hydrostatic Pressures

Atmospheric	Intraocular
760 mmHg	775 mmHg
0 mmHg	15 mmHg

Absolute Pressure

Relative Pressure

Trans-Corneal
Pressure Difference
15mmHg

environment. More properly IOP could be referred to as the transcorneal pressure difference (TCPD). For example, if a patient at sea level has a GAT or transcorneal pressure difference of 15 by GAT, the absolute IOP is 775 mmHg (760 + 15 = 775 mmHg) (see Fig. 5.1).

Diving into a deep-sea environment will cause an increase in the ambient pressure acting on the body. How these changes in ambient pressure affect the body depends on the anatomy of the organs in question. A fluid-filled organ or solid organ will not change in size as the pressure changes because fluids are not compressible. A gas-filled space with elastic walls, however, will change in size and possibly shape. This is due to Boyle's law, which states that the volume of a certain quantity of gas is inversely proportional to the absolute pressure, assuming the temperature remains the same. As an example, a balloon filled with gas at sea level would shrink to one-half its size at a depth of 33 ft. This law is important to divers, as most tissue spaces in the body that contain gas have limited capacity to alter their shape, especially the lungs and middle ear. Therefore, one must add gas to the middle ear on descent to prevent it from collapsing and exhale on ascent to avoid damaging lung tissue. Damage to tissues due to changes in pressure is called barotrauma.

Another applicable principle is described by Henry's Law, which states that the amount of gas that will dissolve in a liquid at a given temperature is directly proportional to the partial pressure of that gas. As a diver descends, the increased pressure causes more nitrogen (the predominant atmospheric gas, comprising 78% of normal air) to enter into solution in his or her tissues than was present at sea level. If enough nitrogen enters the tissues, and the diver ascends too quickly, the excess gas will not have a chance to be eliminated gradually by the lungs. The gas will come out of solution and a gas phase, or bubbles, will form in the blood and body tissues. These bubbles can result in decompression sickness (DCS), also known as "the bends," and will be discussed in greater detail later in the chapter.

Refractive Changes in Water

Two-thirds of the refractive power of the eye is generated by the air-tear film interface. When submerged underwater without a face mask, this interface is changed to water-tear film, and the refractive power of the eye changes dramatically. This change in interface causes approximately five to six diopter hyperopic shift, which is responsible for the blurring of objects when underwater [10].

By wearing a pair of goggles or face mask, the air-tear film interface is restored, and the induced hyperopia is eliminated. However, the light that is traveling toward the eye will be refracted away from the normal as it exits the water and enters the air inside the face mask. This refraction of light will cause the object being viewed to be magnified by approximately 30% and appear closer than it actually is [7, 20].

Refractive Correction Underwater

For persons who need refractive correction while underwater, two options exist: contact lenses and prescription face masks. Soft contact lenses are the preferred lenses to be worn if needed for diving, as hard PMMA lenses can result in corneal edema [5–7, 11, 13]. The edema is due to the formation of nitrogen bubbles in the tear film, which interferes with normal tear physiology and causes epithelial edema [16, 17, 21]. When contact lenses are not an option, prescription face mask lenses provide another alternative. The prescription should be ground into the face mask, as lenses that are bonded onto the faceplate can eventually be displaced as the bonding material is eroded.

Numerous studies have shown that a hyperopic shift, sometimes severe and even permanent, can occur with high-altitude exposure after incisional keratorefractive surgery (see Mader's chapter in this volume). Since part of the effect may be attributable to decreased atmospheric pressure in addition to hypoxia, the potential effect of increased pressure after refractive procedures has been studied in small cohorts of patients. When two subjects (four eyes) who were >1 year out from bilateral radial keratotomy (RK) were exposed to 3 atm in a hyperbaric chamber for 1 h, no changes in keratometry, cycloplegic refraction, and corneal pachymetry were found immediately post-exposure (Peters:1999vo). Additionally, subjects post-LASIK, photorefractive keratectomy (PRK), and RK exhibited no clinically significant change in manifest refraction or best-corrected visual acuity during a simulated dive to 99 FSW (4 atm) in a hyperbaric chamber.

Light Transmission

As light travels through water, it is attenuated by both scattering and absorption. [12] As depth increases, the amount of available light decreases, and the water becomes progressively darker. Even in the clearest waters, only about 20% of incident light reaches a depth of 33 FSW and only 1% reaches 260 FSW [7]. During the day and in clear water, sufficient light for unaided vision is to a depth of approximately 400 FSW [18].

Color Vision

The deep-sea environment can also affect our perception of colors. As the visible light passes through increasing depths of water, selected wavelengths of light are absorbed. Clear water has a maximum transparency of a wavelength of 480 nm, which is near the blue end of the spectrum [7]. Longer wavelengths, such as red and yellow, are absorbed first. Red is usually not seen below 30 ft, and yellow disappears around 75 ft. Below 100 ft only blue and green colors remain without the use of artificial light [18]. Red colors at this depth are then perceived as black [20]. The use of photography or hand-held lights allows for objects to be seen in their actual color at these depths.

Surgical Considerations

Special circumstances exist for patients who have recently undergone ophthalmologic surgery and will be exposed to the increased pressures of the deep sea. Individuals who have had recent surgery must ensure all incisions are healed, as it is possible for pathogens in the environment to enter through the wounds. This could potentially lead to endophthalmitis or other unwanted complications. There are no specific recommendations for participation in diving after eye surgery, and in this situation, adherence to the surgeon's advice about sports after eye surgery should be followed. Data suggest that current small-incision cataract surgery techniques, especially with a scleral tunnel approach, maintain IOP within 30 min after surgery and would not allow fluid ingress or egress thereafter. Mask pressure equilibration (see below) would be particularly important shortly after intraocular surgery, since a negative pressure environment in the mask could draw aqueous and/or vitreous out through any weak area in the healed incision. However, no reports of such occurrences have been published to date, suggesting this concern may be only theoretic. Similarly, while the US Navy considered radial keratotomy (RK) a disqualifier for service, no corneal rupture or wound dehiscence has been reported in recreational divers after RK.

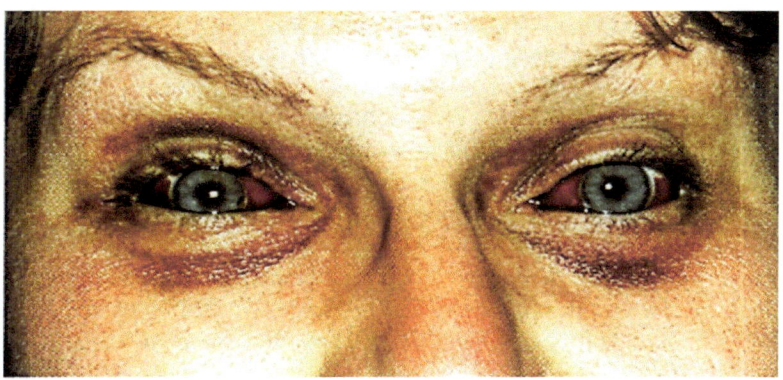

Fig. 5.2 Once a face mask or goggle is placed over the eye, an air chamber is developed that can interact with the eye and ocular adnexa. As a diver descends, this air chamber develops a negative pressure relative to the surroundings, and the eye and surrounding tissues are drawn toward the goggle or mask. This phenomenon has been termed "mask squeeze." If the negative pressure gradient is high enough, it can result in marked edema and ecchymosis of the lids or a subconjunctival hemorrhage

Gas Precautions While Diving

As noted above, solid- or fluid-filled objects maintain a constant shape and size under various pressures. This is true for the eye as well as it is filled with noncompressible aqueous and vitreous. Once a face mask or goggle is placed over the eye, an air chamber is developed that can interact with the eye and ocular adnexa. As a diver descends, this air chamber develops a negative pressure relative to the surroundings, and the eye and surrounding tissues are drawn toward the goggle or mask (Fig. 5.2). This phenomenon has been termed "mask squeeze." If the negative pressure gradient is high enough, it can result in marked edema and ecchymosis of the lids or a subconjunctival hemorrhage. Although these changes can have a very dramatic outward appearance and may cause the patient anxiety and distress, they typically resolve over hours to days with no permanent consequences (Fig. 5.2). Rare instances of orbital subperiosteal hemorrhage also have been described in association with inadequate mask pressure equalization. In order to prevent the negative pressure buildup, positive pressure must be added to this space. The diver can do this by simply blowing air through their nose to add air to the chamber. Because of this, only face masks should be worn for diving, as it is not possible to add air while diving with goggles that just cover the eyes. When the diver ascends, the air in the face mask or goggles will expand. This usually does not cause a problem, as the expanding gas will easily escape from beneath the mask edge where it contacts the skin.

Patients who have intraocular gas bubbles must be extremely careful to avoid large and sudden environmental pressure changes. This includes flying and deep-sea diving. Expanding gas with decreasing pressure, as with increasing altitude in an aircraft cabin or ascent during a dive, may cause intraocular pressure (IOP) elevation as the vitreous cavity expands, while the reverse with hypotony and potential ocular collapse can occur during rapid descent or a controlled underwater dive. The change in IOP is not linear and does not always follow predictions based on volume shifts based on Boyle's law because of anatomic changes such as choroidal volume shifts and ciliary body rotation that also occur. Animal studies in aircraft (LINCOFF) showed that the absolute intraocular pressure decreased after gas expansion during ascent, and this effect was attributed to changes in choroidal volume as well as increased aqueous outflow facility. Scleral buckling may damp the IOP rise associated with gas expansion, as demonstrated by Noble and colleagues in the eyes of 12 patients with partial (10%) gas bubbles (six eyes with scleral buckling) evaluated in a hypobaric chamber in which pressure was reduced to approximately 8000 ft above sea level to simulate commercial air travel. Peak IOP averaged 20 mmHg in the scleral buckle eyes and 32 mmHg in eyes without a buckle.

When rabbits with intraocular gas were placed in a hyperbaric chamber to a depth of 33 FSW (2 atm), the IOP fell from a baseline average 20 mmHg to zero and remained at this level until ascent began. During depressurization and return to 1 atm, the IOP in all subjects rose to over 60 mmHg. This IOP rise occurred even with a brief (60 s) bottom time and subsequent ascent. The IOP spike was attributed to anterior ciliary body rotation from choroidal engorgement with hypotony and obstruction of aqueous outflow as the gas bubble re-expanded. A patient undergoing hyperbaric oxygen therapy for ischemic optic neuropathy while a gas bubble was in the eye exhibited similar findings, with IOP increasing to 50 mmHg at 1 atm after reaching 0 mmHg during exposure to 3 atm. Gross collapse of the eye was not noted at maximal depth. After the dive, slit-lamp examination showed anterior chamber shallowing that remitted as IOP returned to normal. A hollow orbital implant, such as a silicone shell, when used for reconstruction after enucleation could suffer a similar collapse upon diving. If an intraocular gas bubble is in place, the pressure-induced changes in the volume of the bubble can result in serious complications including retinal, uveal, or vitreal hemorrhage or partial collapse of the globe.

Decompression Sickness and Arterial Gas Embolism

As discussed above in Henry's Law, when the body experiences a rapid reduction in ambient pressure, such as moving from deep underwater to the surface, inert gas dissolved in the tissues may come out of solution as bubbles and can form in the body tissues and blood. When these bubbles result in clinical signs or symptoms, the condition is called decompression sickness (DCS).

Sir Robert Boyle first noted ocular involvement in DCS in 1670 when he observed gas bubbles in the anterior chamber of the eye of a viper, which had been experimentally exposed to increased pressure [2]. The incidence of ocular symptoms in patients with DCS is between 7% and 12% and includes nystagmus, diplopia, visual field defects, scotomas, homonymous hemianopsia, orbicularis oculi pain, cortical blindness, convergence insufficiency, optic neuropathy, and central retinal artery occlusion [3, 8, 9, 15, 19]. Most of these ocular symptoms are due to ischemic trauma to the brain or other neural tissue, although it is possible for gas bubbles to form in any ocular tissue. It is exceptionally rare for isolated vision loss from ischemia to occur without other neurological symptoms or findings.

Arterial gas embolism (AGE) is another disorder in which intravascular bubble formation occurs. Rapid ascent causes gas expansion inside the alveoli and alveolar rupture, and the gas bubbles that are formed then enter the pulmonary venous system. From there they enter the heart and then the systemic circulation, where they can disrupt the blood flow to vital organs, including the brain and eye. Patients can present with sudden onset of unconsciousness, motor and/or sensory deficits, hemianopsias, or central retinal artery occlusions. Intravascular gas microbubbles also may form with ascent as decreasing pressure forces gas out of solution. A case report of central retinal artery occlusion in a diver after breathing compressed air during a training scuba dive in a swimming pool demonstrates that undersea pressure may not be necessary for tiny gas emboli to form.

Microembolus formation may be the cause of retinal and choroidal infarcts that have been described in recreational divers, and fluorescein angiography in a cohort of 84 divers showed a number of retinal vascular and retinal pigment epithelial changes that were characteristic of ischemic injury. However, a subsequent report of ocular and retinal findings in 55 Royal Navy divers and 24 non-diving matched controls found no such association between diving history and retinal vascular changes. Following safe diving practices likely prevents retinal ischemia from occurring. Nonetheless, animal studies have captured photographically the presence of retinal vascular microbubbles during rapid ascent from 6 atm pressure, showing that under the appropriate conditions, gas bubble formation and subsequent ischemia may occur.

Treatment of DCS consists of recompression to 60 FSW or deeper and hyperbaric oxygen breathing. Most patients with DCS who are treated properly have resolution of symptoms following treatment. Management of AGE is similar to that for DCS, with emergent recompression and hyperbaric oxygen therapy indicated in all cases. Outcomes of AGE are dependent upon the location and duration of the AGE.

Intraocular Pressure and the Deep-Sea Environment

A patient who enters the deep-sea environment experiences an increase in ambient pressure on their whole body, including the eye. This causes an increase in pressure inside the eye. If the intraocular pressure becomes elevated, why is it that divers don't get optic nerve damage from increased pressure? Certainly the pressure is elevated enough. At a depth of just 33 ft underwater, the ambient pressure is twice that of sea level measuring at 1520 mmHg and the IOP will increase in a similar fashion. For comparison, the ambient pressure in Denver, CO with an elevation of 5280 ft is approximately 640 mmHg. Clearly, the issue is not the absolute pressure

Fig. 5.3 Hydrostatic pressures at sea level and underwater. Note that as the diver moves into the water the various pressures increase, but the transcorneal and translaminar pressure differences remain the same

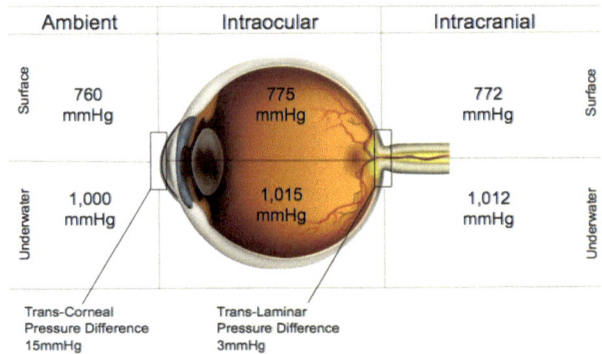

inside the eye, but likely it is the difference between the intraocular pressure and the cerebrospinal fluid pressure (CSFp) immediately posterior to the optic nerve. This is known as the translaminar pressure difference (TLPD) and is similar to the TCPD noted above. Studies have shown that this difference between IOP and CSFp may play a role in development of glaucoma [1, 14]. Saturation divers provide an excellent example for demonstrating how important the TLPD is. These divers spend a prolonged period of time in the deep-sea environment to complete various tasks in order to avoid the lengthy decompression after the dive mission. They are capable of working at a depth of 800 ft and can have absolute intraocular pressures of over 19,000 mmHg. They may remain at these depths for 30 days and do not have any symptoms of glaucomatous optic neuropathy [4, 20]. As the diver moves deeper and deeper, the ambient pressure increases, placing increased pressure on the body and the eye equally. Therefore, the balance between intraocular pressure and CSFp is maintained, and the optic nerve is not damaged (Fig. 5.3).

Summary

In summary, entering the deep-sea environment has multiple effects on the eye. Refractive optics, color, and light transmission are all affected. Serious consequences can result from diving with intraocular gas present, and patients must be cautioned against entering the deep sea if they have a gas bubble present. Decompression sickness and arterial gas embolism are also serious complications that can result from deep-sea diving. Finally, although the intraocular pressure increases with increasing depth, the CSFp also increases, maintaining the TLPD and protecting the eye from glaucomatous damage.

Compliance with Ethical Requirements Michael Greenwood and John Berdahl declare that they have no conflict of interest. No human or animal studies were carried out by the authors for this chapter.

Conflict of Interest Michael Greenwood and John Berdahl declare that they have no conflict of interest.

Informed Consent No human studies were carried out by the authors for this article.

Animal Studies No animal studies were carried out by the authors for this article.

References

1. Berdahl JP, Allingham R, Johnson DH. Cerebrospinal fluid pressure is decreased in primary open-angle glaucoma. Ophthalmology. 2008;115:763–8. 68
2. Butler FK. Decompression sickness. In: Gold DH, Weingeist TA, editors. The eye in systemic disease. Philadelphia: JB Lippincott; 1990. p. 469–71.
3. Butler FK. Decompression sickness presenting as optic neuropathy. Aviat Space Environ Med. 1991;62:346–50.
4. Butler FK. Diving and hyperbaric ophthalmology. Surv Ophthalmol. 1995;39(5):347–66.
5. Cotter J. Soft contact lens testing on fresh water SCUBA divers. Contact Lens. 1981; 7:323–6.
6. Davis JC. Medical evaluation for diving. In: Bore AA, Davis JC, editors. Diving medicine. 2nd ed. Philadelphia: WB Saunders; 1990. p. 296.
7. Edmonds C, Lowry C, Pennefather J. Diving and subaquatic medicine. 3rd ed. Oxford: Butterworth-Heinemann; 1992.
8. Elliott DH, Moon RE. Manifestations of the decompression disorders. In: Bennett PB, Elliott DH, editors. The physiology and medicine of diving. 4th ed. London: WB Saunders; 1993. p. 481–505.
9. Hart BL, Dutka AJ, Flynn ET. Pain-only decompression sickness affecting the orbicularis oculi. Undersea Biomed Res. 1986;13:461–3.
10. Hunter DG, West CE. Last minute optics: a concise review of optics, refraction, and contact lenses. 2nd ed. Slack; 2010. Thorofare, NJ.
11. Josephson JE, Caffery BE. Contact lens considerations in surface and subsurface aqueous environments. Optom Vis Sci. 1991;68:2–11.
12. Kinney JS. Human underwater vision: physiology and physics. Bethesda: Undersea and Hyperbaric Society; 1985. p. 41–9.
13. Mebane GY, McIver NKI. Fitness to dive. In: Bennett PB, Elliott DH, editors. The physiology and medicine of diving. 4th ed. London: WB Saunders; 1993. p. 59–60.
14. Ren RJ, Jonas JB, Tian GG, et al. Cerebrospinal fluid pressure in glaucoma A prospective study. Ophthalmology. 2010;117:259–66.
15. Rivera JC. Decompression sickness among divers – an analysis of 935 cases. Mil Med. 1964;129:314–34.
16. Simon DR, Bradley ME. Corneal edema in divers wearing hard contact lenses. Am J Ophthalmol. 1978;85:462–4.
17. Simon DR, Bradley ME. Adverse effects of contact lens wear during decompression. JAMA. 1980;244:1213–4.
18. Somers LH. Diving physics. In: Bore AA, Davis JC, editors. Diving medicine. 2nd ed. Philadelphia: WB Saunders; 1990. p. 15–6.

19. Summitt JK, Berghage TE. Review of diving accident reports, 1968. US Navy Experimental Diving Unit research report. 1970. p. 11–70. San Diego, CA.
20. US Navy Diving Manual. Commander naval sea systems command publication 0910-LP-106-0957. Washington, DC: US Government Press; 2011. Revision 6.
21. Wilmshurst P. Retinal changes, gas bubbles, and diving (letter). Lancet. 1989;8635:438.

Chapter 6
Lessons from Animals in Extreme Environments

Michael J. Mines and Christopher O. Ochieng

Accommodation in Air and Water

The human eye is poorly adapted to fine visual acuity in an aquatic environment. The air-cornea interface accounts for approximately 66% of the eye's non-accommodated refractive power. When immersed in water, the anterior corneal dioptric power of over 40 diopters (D) is largely neutralized, leaving the eye with severe hyperopic defocus [5]. Even maximal accommodation is unable replace the lost corneal refractive power. Divers learn that to overcome this effect, goggles or a mask must be worn which restores the air-corneal interface and introduces a flat, zero refractive power boundary between the water and goggles/mask [6].

As one would expect, fish are well suited for underwater vision. Without a need for refractive curvature and likely to reduce drag in water, their corneas are relatively flattened [7]. Refraction is accomplished by a relatively powerful lens which tends to be spherical in shape and is further enhanced by a gradient of refractive index [14]. Rather than a deforming lens as in humans, in fish, accommodation is generally performed by the physical movement of the lens relative to the retina.

Between these extremes, some animals occupy an amphibious ecological niche that requires useful visual acuity both while in air and submerged. Typically hunters, these animals live on land but locate, pursue, and capture prey while underwater. Interestingly they have adapted various different methods to overcome the induced hyperopia caused by the loss of corneal power when submerged. One type of ocular modification is found in penguins. Contrary to initial thought that these birds were

M.J. Mines, MD, DVM (✉) • C.O. Ochieng, MD
Madigan Army Medical Center, Department of Surgery, Ophthalmology Service,
Tacoma, WA, USA
e-mail: michael.j.mines.mil@mail.mil

© Springer International Publishing AG 2017   83
P.S. Subramanian (ed.), *Ophthalmology in Extreme Environments*,
Essentials in Ophthalmology, DOI 10.1007/978-3-319-57600-8_6

adapted to aquatic vision and therefore myopic in air, newer studies show that they are actually emmetropic in both environments [11]. Observations made by Howland and Sivak studying four different penguin species (Magellanic, King, Gentoo, Rockhoppers) using photokeratoscopy showed that, like fish, they possess relatively flat corneal curvatures. In Rockhoppers and Magellanic penguins, corneal power was approximately 30D with axial lengths of 23 mm and 27 mm, respectively. While in aerial birds like the pigeon corneal radius is about one half globe radius indicative of more corneal power, in penguins corneal radii approximate globe radii. Despite flatter corneas, photorefractive testing in air demonstrated that these penguins remained emmetropic. When entering water, however, even this reduced corneal power is lost. Yet similar testing of the birds in water showed that the lost dioptric power of the cornea is taken up by an exaggerated accommodative ability. The flatter corneas come at a cost in that penguins have decreased monocular visual fields compared to nonaquatic birds. This technique of flattened corneas and powerful spherical lenses as a method of underwater vision is not unique to penguins and fish. Marine mammals also exhibit varying degrees of both in nature [8, 28].

Other bird species that visually locate and capture prey underwater possess corneas of the curved terrestrial model. Separate from birds that spot prey from the air and immediately secure their target on entering the water with bill strikes, plunges, or talons, pursuit diving birds identify prey while flying above the water but actively pursue fish by swimming once below the surface [16]. These birds like cormorants and gannets have relatively high corneal curvature and resultant dioptric power in air ranging from 40 to 60 D [13, 16]. To account for the immediate loss of corneal power underwater, both species are able to accommodate within 40–80 ms and to a degree where they exhibit underwater myopia as they visualize near targets. In earlier experiments with enucleated merganser and goldeneye duck eyes, similar high corneal curvatures and neutralizing accommodative ability were found [27].

While humans are at a significant disadvantage in terms of unaided submerged visual acuity when compared to many aquatically adapted animals, recent studies reveal that at least modest gains are possible and in fact are being employed today. The Moken, a tribe of sea nomads of Southeast Asia, live off the ocean. Their children engage in visually oriented tasks, collecting food and shells underwater, without the aid of masks [5]. When compared to European children of similar age, Moken children demonstrated twice the visual acuity underwater (6.06 ± 0.59 cycles per degree (c/d) vs 2.95 ± 0.13 c/d). Researchers determined that when submerged, Moken children manifested significantly smaller pupils, improving depth of field. In addition, they calculated that Moken children maximally accommodated while underwater further increasing aquatic visual acuity. These findings were specific to water vision; in air they found no difference between the groups. In a following study, Gislén et al. went on to determine whether non-Moken children could be trained to perform as well as Moken children underwater [6]. That investigation revealed these underwater vision results are not specific to Moken, but non-Moken children can learn to improve submerged acuity by applying similar techniques.

Finally the four-eyed fish (*Anableps anableps*) employs a truly remarkable method of combined aerial and submarine vision. Instead of adapting to the dramatic

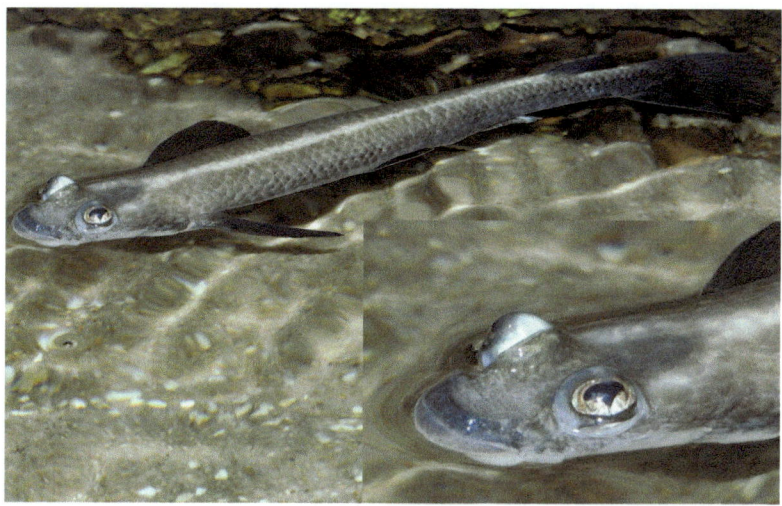

Fig. 6.1 Photograph of a four-eyed fish (*Anableps anableps*). Inset demonstrates aerial and submerged cornea (Adapted from source: https://commons.wikimedia.org/wiki/File:Anableps_anableps_qtl1.jpg. Original author: Quartl. Used as licensed under the Creative Commons Attribution-Share Alike 3.0 Unported license)

change of moving between environments, this fish swims at the water's surface with half of each eye above and the other half below the water line [7]. A pigmented band extends across the cornea at the air-water interface. The dorsal, aerial cornea is curved while the submerged cornea is relatively shallow. The pupil has two apertures – creating two visual pathways. Yet despite separate pathways, each eye contains only a single elliptical lens. Light originating from above encounters a thinner, less curved lens; light from the aquatic environment, without the benefit of corneal power, encounters an axis of the lens that is more spherical and refractive (Figs. 6.1 and 6.2). With this optical arrangement, the ventral and dorsal retinal areas receive light from different environments, downwelling and upwelling, respectively. The specialization does not end there. Opsin gene evaluation indicates that the ventral and dorsal retinas in *Anableps* differ in opsin expression, corresponding and optimized to wavelengths from each source [20].

Pupil Morphology

Pupil morphology in the animal world is both elegant and complex. While we may be most familiar with the round pupils of primates, pupils manifest a variety of shapes. Pupils are configured as vertically oriented slits, horizontally slit, crescent shaped, and even "W" shaped. In addition the aperture is typically open but may be variably occluded with an operculum. Each configuration endows the owner with certain optical characteristics advantageous to its ecological niche.

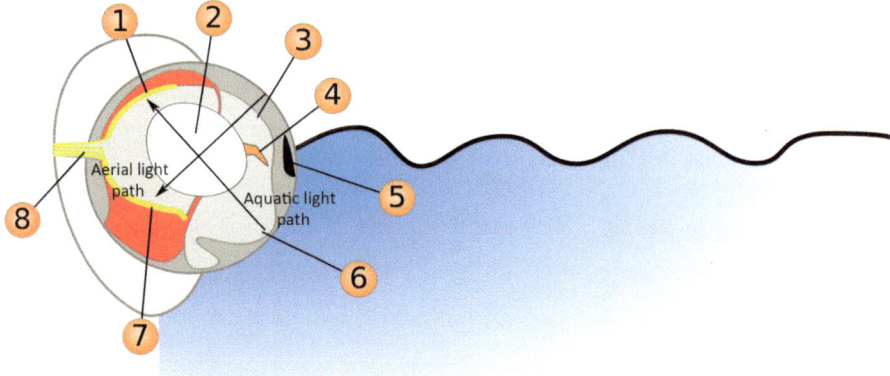

Fig. 6.2 Diagram of the eye of a four-eyed fish (*Anableps anableps*): *1* dorsal retina (views submerged scene), *2* lens with greater power along the aquatic light path axis, *3* dorsal pupil, *4* iris, *5* tissue band, *6* ventral (submerged) pupil, *7* ventral retina (views aerial scene), and *8* optic nerve (Adapted from source https://commons.wikimedia.org/wiki/File:Schema_Auge_Vieraugenfisch. svg. Original author: Sgbeer. Used under the terms of the GNU Free Documentation License, Version 1.2 and licensed under the Creative Commons Attribution-Share Alike 3.0 Unported, 2.5 Generic, 2.0 Generic and 1.0 Generic license)

Humans and other animals with round pupils balance the benefits of visual acuity with the need for light collection. Given the retina's photoreceptor architecture, in ample lighting conditions, a pupil size of approximately 2–3 mm maximizes the optical system's resolution potential [14]. Smaller pupil size induces diffraction, and a larger size leads to chromatic and spherical aberration, both deteriorating visual resolution. However, as ambient light decreases, visual acuity declines due to photon noise and the disadvantages of a larger pupil are outweighed by increased light capture.

In the animal kingdom, it is noted that certain predators possess vertically slit pupils [2]. Animals as diverse as cats, certain geckos and snakes have vertical pupils, and while dissimilar in many respects, they all share an ambush hunting style and forage in limited light [3]. These vertical pupils are much more efficient at reducing light passage. Whereas humans can change pupil area 16-fold between light and dark conditions, the domestic cat (*Felis catus*) is capable of a 135-fold change, or ten times that of humans [14] (see Fig. 6.3). The Tokay gecko (*Gekko gecko*), a nocturnal hunter, possesses a pupil that in scotopic conditions is round. In daylight however its vertical pupil margins abut, completely closing the pupil aperture saved for two small notches (See Fig. 6.4). The resulting pupil measures 0.1 mm, a 300-fold decrease in pupil area [4]. While in a human, a pupil of that size would result in significant diffraction and degraded resolution, the shorter length of the gecko eye coupled with its retinal photoreceptor spacing permits such a small pupil to be optically functional.

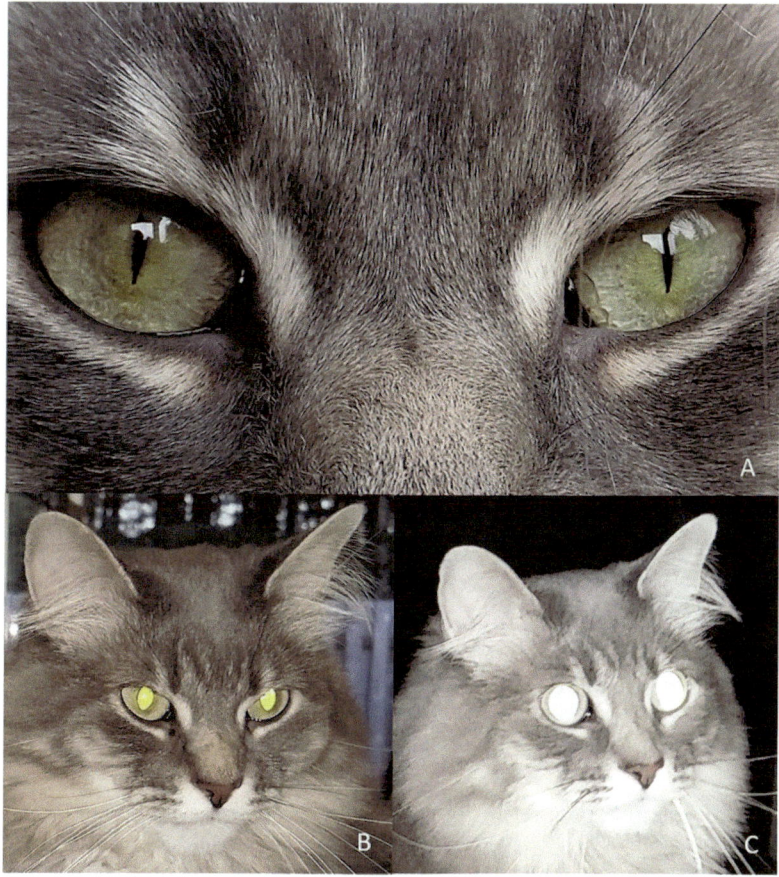

Fig. 6.3 Domestic cat (*Felis catus*). (**A**) Vertically slit pupils typical of the domestic cat in photopic conditions. (**B**) Mid-dilated pupils demonstrating *yellow* tapetal reflex. (**C**) Dilated pupils. Taken in very dim illumination to demonstrate pupillary dilation, the tapetal reflexes appear nearly white in this image (Source – author MJM. Subject: Alice the cat.)

Authors have theorized why such a dramatic ability to limit retinal illumination exists in these animals. To be sure pupil constriction does protect the retina from sudden illumination changes. And as described above, optimizing pupil size strikes a balance between diffraction and aberration at various light levels. An additional reason is retinal sensitivity. This characteristic is dependent on several factors including photoreceptor (PR) spacing, PR alignment relative to incident light, tapetal reflection (see Section – Tapetum Lucidum below), and post PR stimulation signal summation. Various animals use some or all of these to maximize retinal sensitivity to light stimulation, and on an order far greater than man. For example, the helmet gecko's retina is 350 times more sensitive compared to a human retina at light levels where the eye can discriminate color [23]. This level of sensitivity is an obvious advantage when hunting in dim illumination, but without a means to limit

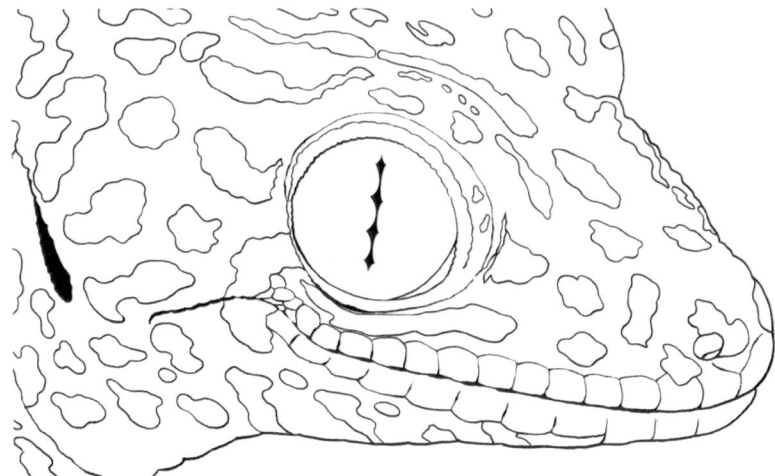

Fig. 6.4 Representative Gecko eye with multi-notched pupil. Public domain (Source: U.S. Geological Survey, Department of the Interior/USGS. The USGS home page is http://www. usgs.gov.)

retinal illumination would render an animal blind at higher light levels. Slit pupils therefore, with their more efficient ability to limit pupil area and light passage, permit useful visual function over a broad range of light intensities.

Another consideration of slit pupils besides pupil area is lens exposure. With round pupils, as pupillary dilation increases, not only is more light permitted into the optical system but more of the peripheral lens is exposed, refracting incident light. In dim light levels, the resulting chromatic aberration may be a necessary trade-off for increased retinal illumination. In animals with a slit pupil, relatively more peripheral lens is inevitably exposed for a given light level. This seemingly induced limitation would be explained if lenses of slit pupil animals corrected for chromatic aberration. In fact Malmström and Kröger investigated the optical systems of terrestrial vertebrates both with and without slit pupils and determined that in every case they studied, the lenses of animals with slit pupils did just that [17]. Described as multifocal lenses, these lenses have gradients of refractive indices allowing various wavelengths to be simultaneously well focused, overcoming chromatic aberration. Multifocal lenses were found not only in species with vertical slit pupils like small felines (cats) and small canines (red fox), but also in those with horizontal slit pupils like sheep, reindeer, elk, and horse. In species examined by the authors having round pupils, nearly all exhibited monofocal lenses, or lenses that did not correct for chromatic aberration. This included large felines like the Siberian tiger (*Panthera tigris altaica*). Interestingly the intermediate felid species Eurasian lynx (*Lynx lynx*) has oval pupils and an intermediate form of lens.

While a slit pupil is advantageous when one has a multifocal lens system, minimizing chromatic aberration cannot be the sole reason for a non-round pupil. The octopus has a horizontally slit pupil yet is color blind [14]. Chromatic defocus would not be noted in this species. Like external color, spot patterns, and contour, a slit pupil may provide camouflage or perhaps not be as noticeable as a round pupil while still maintaining visual function [7]. This may be at least one of the reasons the cuttlefish has a W-shaped pupil in bright illumination. The dolphin pupil possesses a dorsal (superior) operculum which shades the inferior retina from the disproportionate amount of light originating from above in marine environments [7]. Similarly the cuttlefish's W-shaped pupil is effective in balancing a vertically uneven light field [18]. Elongated or complex-shaped pupils also appear to convey visual advantage in terms of contrast, pinhole effect, depth of field, and enhancing vertical or horizontal contour depending on pupil orientation [2, 18, 23].

Tapetum Lucidum

The human eye functions effectively over a wide range of illumination. Spanning luminance levels from bright sunlight to less than nighttime star light, human sensitivity extends between 10^{20} and 10^{10} photons per second per square meter [14]. In terms of absolute sensitivity, however, we like other diurnal species are poorly suited for nocturnal visual endeavors. Many animals that typically spend much of their active periods in dim light exhibit sensitivities greater than man. Various optical and anatomic methods account for this increased sensitivity including photoreceptor size and spacing, maximum pupil diameter, and overall eye size. An interesting additional ocular structure, common even in our household pets, is the tapetum lucidum.

One of the better known examples of the tapetum lucidum [Latin: "bright/shining tapestry or carpet"] is found in the domestic cat (*Felis catus*) and is responsible for the phenomenon often called "eye shine" (see Fig. 6.3) [15, 21]. It functions as a biological mirror, reflecting incident light not initially captured back through the photoreceptors, providing a second opportunity for photon-photoreceptor stimulation and thereby increasing light sensitivity [19]. Nearly all primates, birds, and rodents, as well as the squirrel and pig, do not possess a tapetum [19, 26]. Yet it appears a tapetum confers some ecological advantage since it is found in a number of species including numerous vertebrates, as well as invertebrate mollusk and arthropods [26, 29]. While the method of its employment varies both in location and how reflectance is accomplished in these animals, the commonality is that the tapetum can result in high reflectance due to a structural arrangement that produces exceedingly efficient constructive interference, theoretically approaching 100% [14]. Blood vessels, cell nuclei, and variation in cell spacing interfere, but this is overcome by making use of multiple layers of the tapetal tissue, improving reflectance by summation [14]. The actual reflective material differs among species but include lipid, guanine crystals, riboflavin, and zinc cysteine [19, 26]. Even melanin and collagen under the correct conditions are transformed to become efficient reflectors.

The three general types of tapeta are a retinal tapetum and two choroidal tapeta, the tapetum cellulosum and tapetum fibrosum. The retinal tapetum is found in various fishes, reptiles like crocodiles and alligators, opossums, and fruit bats [26]. It is subdivided as non-occlusible or occlusible. The reflecting medium is composed of lipid, guanine, or melanin. The retinal tapetum, occlusible type is found in some fish and is responsible for variation in tapetal reflectance. Unlike the static or non-occlusible tapetum, in the occlusible form, the reflecting media migrate within the retinal pigment epithelium (RPE) toward or away from the vitreous depending on illumination level. This exposes or masks the reflecting tapetum in dim or bright light, respectively [19]. In other fish species instead of pigment migration, tapetal reflectance is blocked by visual cell movement and migration of RPE processes. The occlusible tapetum is less efficient and thought to primarily benefit the animal by reducing "eye shine"-mediated detection.

Both types of choroidal tapeta are interspaced just external to the choriocapillaris and internal to the remaining choroidal stroma. The RPE overlying the tapetal region has no melanin granules permitting light to both pass through and be reflected back toward the retinal photoreceptors [30]. The area over which the tapetum is present varies between species but is not typically complete, frequently occupying a swath most prominent in the dorsal retina and tapering with a covering RPE layer more peripherally [19, 29, 30]. The cellular variant, the choroidal tapetum cellulosum, is found in many mammalian carnivores, like cats and dogs, and cartilaginous (sharks, dogfishes) and lobe-fined (lungfishes) fish [19, 26]. The cat possesses one of the most refined cellular tapeta, consisting of rodlets containing riboflavin and zinc cysteine and arranged in a precise hexagonal lattice pattern [19]. The remarkable structural organization, and uniform thickness and spacing tolerance per layer, provides a highly efficient quarter wavelength interference reflector [14].

Unlike the cellular tapetum, which requires a secondary spectral substance, the choroidal tapetum fibrosum accomplishes reflection by the arrangement and orientation of its collagen fibers. Just external to the choriocapillaris, the collagen fibrils are aligned parallel to the retina and at a right angle to incident light [29, 30]. Like the cellular tapetum, the collagen is arranged in a hexagonal array with regular spacing [19]. Fibrous tapeta are noted in ungulates (cow, goats, sheep, and horses) and cetacea (whales, dolphins).

Because tapetal reflectance is dependent on the diameter and spacing of the reflective structures, it is wavelength specific [32]. Hence, species typically have a predominant tapetal "eye shine" color. However, it appears that the Arctic reindeer has developed a useful adaptation resulting not only in a variable colored tapetal reflex but one that changes in relation to available ambient light conditions. Arctic reindeer experience extreme changes in photic conditions with periods of complete daylight in summer and extended periods of twilight to near complete darkness in winter. During winter months, lighting becomes diffuse and is relatively shifted to shorter wavelengths [10]. Hogg et al. determined that these reindeers' visual sensitivity extends into the near UV range. Interestingly, Stokkan et al. observed that in summer, these animals exhibit a golden tapetal reflex with high reflectance; in winter however the reflex is diffuse and deep blue [32]. They determined the shift to a blue reflection in winter animals depended on a change in collagen spacing associated with persistent pupillary dilation and increased intraocular pressure

(IOP). The elevated IOP they postulated, resulted in increased collagen compression and reflection of shorter wavelengths corresponding to the available ambient winter light. While visual acuity declines, the blue shift increases tangential scatter of reflected light and improves retinal sensitivity in the low illumination seasons.

Raptor Vision

One of the truly spectacular displays in nature is the attack dive, or stoop, of a falcon (see – http://video.nationalgeographic.com/video/falcon_peregrine_velocity). While difficult to accurately measure, a peregrine falcon in the wild is estimated to be able to reach speeds of 100 meters per second (m/s) or 220 miles per hour (mph), and in fact a trained peregrine falcon has been recorded at over 240 mph. [9, 33]. While these top speeds may be brief or used sparingly, velocities ranging from 80 to 150 mph (40–70 m/s) appear common and equate to traveling nearly the length of a football field every second [1, 35, 36]. To both achieve and maintain such velocities, it is critical that these birds maximize their body aerodynamics to minimize drag and instability. Yet speed is not the raptor's only remarkable characteristic. Tucker noted that falcons frequently identified prey, robin-sized birds, at distances of 1500 m or more [36]. What characteristics permit raptors to locate and identify prey over great distances and visually track that prey while moving at such high rates of speed?

Raptors like the peregrine falcon can assume an efficient aerodynamic shape which permits high-velocity dives. At these speeds maintenance of optimal configuration is important, and even small changes in positioning can impact overall performance. In fact by changing shape away from a maximally efficient aerodynamic configuration, the animal can intentionally induce drag, slowing their descent. It is clear then that minimizing unwanted drag is critical. A conflict however could develop between maintaining an aerodynamic shape and maintaining visual fixation on their targeted prey. Raptors only minimally rotate their eyes within their orbits. When stationary or in gliding (slow) flight, fixation is primarily accomplished with head movements [34]. Similar head movements at high speeds will induce drag and torque - drag which slows the animal and torque which will require a compensatory position change to counter act it, further reducing velocity.

Birds of prey overcome this potential reduction in performance by utilizing two distinct foveae per retina. The shallow fovea is located more temporally and is 15° off the center head axis (see Fig. 6.5), whereas the deep fovea is positioned nasally with a "line of sight" corresponding to approximately 45° externally off of midline [34]. Studies in Chilean eagles demonstrate retinal receptor density is highest in the deep fovea with a second lower peak in the shallow fovea [12]. Spectral domain optical coherence tomography of the retina in another raptor species, the short-tailed hawk, reveals a deep fovea morphologically similar to humans and a second distinct foveal region with a shallower pit [24]. These anatomic findings correspond well with observational studies [34]. Several raptor species behaviorally assume one

Fig. 6.5 Diagram of raptor skull demonstrating relative positions of shallow and deep foveae (Author: MJM. Source: Various)

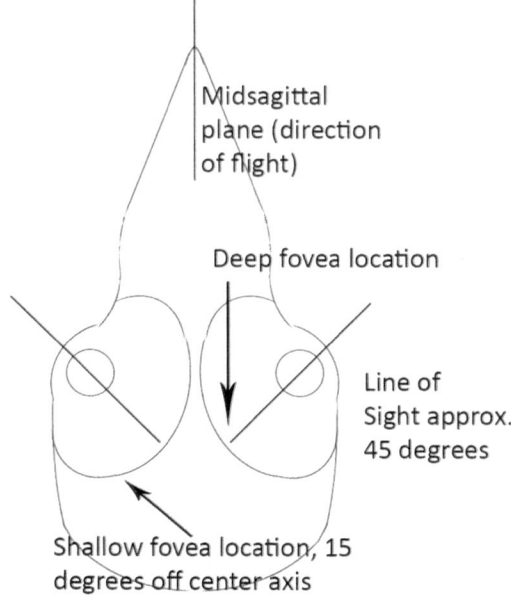

Midsagittal plane (direction of flight)

Deep fovea location

Line of Sight approx. 45 degrees

Shallow fovea location, 15 degrees off center axis

of three head positions when fixating a target. At distances up to 8 m, they view an object straight ahead, corresponding to the shallow foveae. At distances between 8 and 21 m, they increasingly view objects of interest from an angle of roughly 45° to the left or right of midline. At distances greater than 40 m, 80% of viewing is performed from this sideways angle.

Both anatomically and behaviorally, then, it appears that raptors like the peregrine falcon have the most acute vision when viewing at an angle of 45° from midline. Maintaining fixation with the deep fovea during a high-speed dive would overcome the drag and torque disadvantage brought on by a head turn. It would not however allow a direct line of flight, but rather a spiral approach would be required. Tucker demonstrated theoretically that, given the speed penalty of a required head turn when following a direct path, a raptor could approach prey in a curved path more efficiently [34]. Observations of wild peregrine falcons revealed in fact they did make use of this technique during the dive phase [36]. Only when nearing the target did their flight path become direct, presumably where bilateral use of the shallow foveae and stereopsis became more beneficial [34].

The great speed advantage exhibited by hawks, falcons, and eagles does require sufficient distance to permit a dive maneuver. That distance also necessitates an optical system capable of fine resolution; falcons have been noted to initiate pursuit of prey measuring roughly 30 cm in width at 1500 m. [36] Humans can resolve approximately 60–70 c/d. Reymond found that the *Aquila* eagle's maximum acuity is between 132 and 143 c/d, or twice as fine as man [22]. This is accomplished in several ways [14]. A raptor's photopic pupil is larger than in a human, decreasing blur due to diffraction. Additionally, the photoreceptors are narrower which

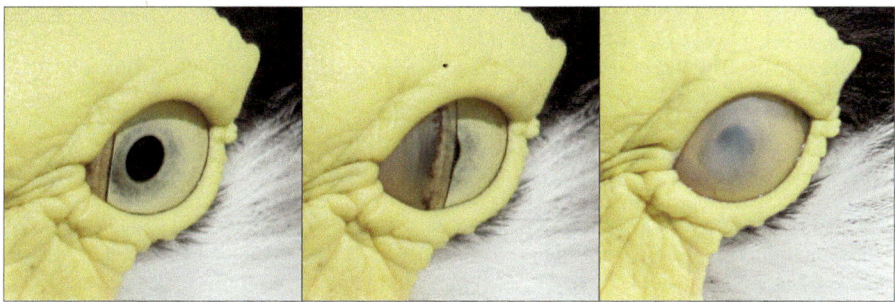

Fig. 6.6 Avian nictitating membrane, in this case a Masked Lapwing, demonstrating its path across the cornea (Author: Toby Hudson. Source: https://en.wikipedia.org/wiki/File:Bird_blink-edit.jpg. Used as licensed under the Creative Commons Attribution-Share Alike 3.0 Unported license)

improves retinal sampling frequency and maximum resolution. Finally, it appears that in these animals the foveal pit functions as a negative lens due to local refractive index differences [31]. Together with the anatomic lens, a telescopic effect is created extending the effective focal length of the eye. The resultant image is therefore magnified, further improving resolution.

Yet even with their finer resolving ability, if the refracting system – cornea, lens, and ocular media – is not clear, the image will be degraded. Humans engaged in high-speed activities like professional open cockpit race drivers and skydivers wear goggles to protect their eyes and maintain corneal clarity. Birds and many other animals possess a nictitating membrane, or third eyelid to perform a similar function (See Fig. 6.6). Containing striated muscle this membrane moves across the cornea maintaining a uniform tear film and clearing collected debris [25]. Specialized feather epithelium appears to line the edge, further assisting.

In all, diving birds of prey are remarkably well adapted to maximizing their physiology to advantage. Coupled with an efficient aerodynamic design, the raptors' exceptional acuity, nictitating membrane and specialized bifoveate retinal architecture enable these creatures to not only function but to excel at the extremes of animal performance, and induce fascination in their less visually acute human watchers.

Compliance with Ethical Requirements Michael Mines and Christopher Ochieng declare we have no conflict of interest. No human or animal studies were carried out by the authors for this article.

References

1. Alerstam T. Radar observations of the stoop of the Peregrine Falcon *Falco peregrinus* and the Goshawk *Accipiter gentilis*. Ibis. 1987;129:267–73.
2. Banks MS, Sprague WW, Schmoll J, et al. Why do animal eyes have pupils of different shapes? Sci Adv. 2015;1(7):e1500391.

3. Brischoux F, Pizzatto L, Shine R. Insights into the adaptive significance of vertical pupil shape in snakes. J Evol Biol. 2010;23(9):1878–85.

4. Denton EJ. The responses of the pupil of Gekko gekko to external light stimulus. J Gen Physiol. 1956;40(2):201–16.

5. Gislén A, Dacke M, Kröger RH, et al. Superior underwater vision in a human population of sea gypsies. Curr Biol. 2003;13(10):833–6.

6. Gislén A, Warrant EJ, Dacke M, et al. Visual training improves underwater vision in children. Vis Res. 2006;46(20):3443–50.

7. González-Martín-Moro J, Gómez-Sanz F, Sales-Sanz A, et al. Pupil shape in the animal kingdom: from the pseudopupil to the vertical pupil. Arch Soc Esp Oftalmol. 2014;89(12):484–94.

8. Hanke FD, Dehnhardt G, Schaeffel F, et al. Corneal topography, refractive state, and accommodation in harbor seals (*Phoca vitulina*). Vis Res. 2006;46(6–7):837–47.

9. Harpole T (2005) Falling with the Falcon. Peregrines think simple thoughts: See food. Fly down. Go fast. Very fast. Air & Space Magazine march 2005. Available via http://www.airspacemag.com/flight-today/falling-with-the-falcon-7491768/?all&no-ist. Accessed 1 June 2016.

10. Hogg C, Neveu M, Stokkan KA, et al. Arctic reindeer extend their visual range into the ultraviolet. J Exp Biol. 2011;214(Pt 12):2014–9.

11. Howland HC, Sivak JG. Penguin vision in air and water. Vis Res. 1984;24(12):1905–9.

12. Inzunza O, Bravo H, Smith RL, et al. Topography and morphology of retinal ganglion cells in Falconiforms: a study on predatory and carrion-eating birds. Anat Rec. 1991;229(2):271–7.

13. Katzir G, Howland HC. Corneal power and underwater accommodation in great cormorants (*Phalacrocorax carbo sinensis*). J Exp Biol. 2003;206(Pt 5):833–41.

14. Land MF, Nilsson DE. Animal Eyes. Oxford: Oxford University Press; 2012.

15. Latin Word Lookup. University of Notre Dame. 2016. http://www.archives.nd.edu/cgi-bin/lookup.pl?stem=tapet&ending=um. Accessed 1 June 2016.

16. Machovsky-Capuska GE, Howland HC, Raubenheimer D, et al. Visual accommodation and active pursuit of prey underwater in a plunge-diving bird: the Australasian gannet. Proc Biol Sci. 2012;279(1745):4118–25.

17. Malmström T, Kröger RH. Pupil shapes and lens optics in the eyes of terrestrial vertebrates. J Exp Biol. 2006;209(Pt 1):18–25.

18. Mäthger LM, Hanlon RT, Håkansson J, et al. The W-shaped pupil in cuttlefish (*Sepia officinalis*): functions for improving horizontal vision. Vis Res. 2013;83:19–24.

19. Ollivier FJ, Samuelson DA, Brooks DE, et al. Comparative morphology of the tapetum lucidum (among selected species). Vet Ophthalmol. 2004;7(1):11–22.

20. Owens GL, Rennison DJ, Allison WT, et al. In the four-eyed fish (*Anableps anableps*), the regions of the retina exposed to aquatic and aerial light do not express the same set of opsin genes. Biol Lett. 2012;8(1):86–9.

21. Perseus Digital Library. Tufts University, Latin Word Study Tool. 2016. http://www.perseus.tufts.edu/hopper/morph?l=lucidum&la=la. Accessed 1 June 2016.

22. Reymond L. Spatial visual acuity of the falcon, *Falco berigora*: a behavioural, optical and anatomical investigation. Vis Res. 1987;27(10):1859–74.

23. Roth LS, Lundström L, Kelber A, et al. The pupils and optical systems of gecko eyes. J Vis. 2009;9(3):27.1–11.

24. Ruggeri M, Major JC Jr, McKeown C, et al. Retinal structure of birds of prey revealed by ultra-high resolution spectral-domain optical coherence tomography. Invest Ophthalmol Vis Sci. 2010;51(11):5789–95.

25. Schwab IR, Maggs D. The falcon's stoop. Br J Ophthalmol. 2004;88(1):4.

26. Schwab IR, Yuen CK, Buyukmihci NC, et al. Evolution of the tapetum. Trans Am Ophthalmol Soc. 2002;100:187–99.

27. Sivak JG, Hildebrand T, Lebert C. Magnitude and rate of accommodation in diving and non-diving birds. Vis Res. 1985;25(7):925–33.

28. Sivak JG, Howland HC, West J, et al. The eye of the hooded seal, *Cystophora cristata*, in air and water. J Comp Physiol A. 1989;165(6):771–7.

29. Shinozaki A, Hosaka Y, Imagawa T, et al. Relationship between distribution of tapetum fibrosum and retinal pigment epithelium in the sheep eye. J Vet Med Sci. 2010;72(2):211–5.
30. Shinozaki A, Takagi S, Hosaka YZ, et al. The fibrous tapetum of the horse eye. J Anat. 2013;223(5):509–18.
31. Snyder AW, Miller WH. Telephoto lens system of falconiform eyes. Nature. 1978;275(5676):127–9.
32. Stokkan KA, Folkow L, Dukes J, et al. Shifting mirrors: adaptive changes in retinal reflections to winter darkness in Arctic reindeer. Proc Biol Sci. 2013;280(1773):20132451.
33. Tucker VA. Gliding flight: speed and acceleration of ideal falcons during diving and pull out. J Exp Biol. 1998;201(Pt 3):403–14.
34. Tucker VA. The deep fovea, sideways vision and spiral flight paths in raptors. J Exp Biol. 2000;203(Pt 24):3745–54.
35. Tucker VA, Cade TJ, Tucker AE. Diving speeds and angles of a gyrfalcon (*Falco rusticolus*). J Exp Biol. 1998;201(Pt 13):2061–70.
36. Tucker VA, Tucker AE, Akers K, et al. Curved flight paths and sideways vision in peregrine falcons (*Falco peregrinus*). J Exp Biol. 2000;203(Pt 24):3755–63.

Chapter 7
Industrial and Military Eye Injuries and Eye Protection Challenges

Arjuna M. Subramanian and Prem S. Subramanian

Introduction

Eye injuries are prevalent in environments with high-velocity particle motion and/ or high temperatures, and injuries range from periocular contusions and burns to corneoscleral lacerations and frank globe ruptures. Although they often are available, protective devices may be unused and/or not mandated. Such environments include heavy industrial settings such as metalworking and welding, in which workers are exposed to threats from sometimes red-hot and fast-moving metal shards, although these risks can be reduced with mandatory safety regimens. Many sports, including lacrosse, baseball, squash, and ice hockey – activities that particularly center around relatively small and hard balls and pucks moving at high speeds – also feature high eye injury rates, usually in the absence (baseball, squash) or inefficacy (ice hockey, lacrosse) of safety equipment.

A survey of serious eye injury occurrence in the United States published in 2000 pronounced the home to be the area of greatest danger, with 41% of all injuries occurring in this environment; industrial settings placed second at 14%, and sports and recreation activities third at 13% [22]. This marked a substantial decrease from

---

Supported in part by an unrestricted grant from Research to Prevent Blindness, Inc. to the Department of Ophthalmology, University of Colorado School of Medicine.

A.M. Subramanian
Department of Ophthalmology, University of Colorado School of Medicine,
1675 Aurora Ct, Mail Stop F731, Aurora, CO 80045, USA

P.S. Subramanian, MD, PhD (✉)
Departments of Ophthalmology, Neurology, and Neurosurgery, University of Colorado School of Medicine, Aurora, CO, USA
e-mail: prem.subramanian@ucdenver.edu

© Springer International Publishing AG 2017
P.S. Subramanian (ed.), *Ophthalmology in Extreme Environments*,
Essentials in Ophthalmology, DOI 10.1007/978-3-319-57600-8_7

the 69.9% injury share for workplace-related incidents reported in a comparable British study from 11 years earlier [20]. Unsurprisingly, the vast majority of all ocular injuries in US analysis, 78%, involved individuals wearing no eye protection, compared to 2% wearing actual safety glasses and 3% with use of any eyewear [22]. Industries requiring welding tasks, including the manufacturing and construction sectors, form a representative and instructive case of the circumstances and prevalence of ocular injuries. According to one analysis, 25% of all workers' compensation claims filed by welders during the year 2000 were related to ocular injuries; by comparison, eye injuries comprised 5% of all injuries to all workers [19]. The most common source of injury was a foreign body such as particulate matter, hot substances or chemicals, which comprised 71.7% of eye injuries. Periocular and corneal burns from either heat and/or UV light were next most frequent at 22.2% [19]. The effect of using protective eyewear could not be determined reliably, as only 14.7–17.6% of claims even mentioned the use (or non-use) of personal protective equipment. Industrial ocular injuries, although frequently minor and not vision threatening, result both in worker anxiety and lost productivity, and the effect of such injuries on worker retention has not been studied. More serious injuries, such as corneal scarring from UV exposure and globe perforation by foreign bodies, also can be prevented but continue to occur nonetheless [27].

Barriers to Change

If the impact of mandating safety equipment can be so marked – reducing the occurrence of eye injuries by as much as a factor of 14.5 in one study of metalworking facilities [3] – how come such measures have not become universal? Obstacles of cost and cultural resistance form the most significant barriers towards increasing the rate of eye protection adoption.

The cultural roadblock is particularly noticeable in industrial settings, likely due at least in part to both sectors' historical association with demonstrable masculinity. In tasks commonly associated with ocular injuries – grinding, welding, drilling, automotive work, and other working-class industries – the index of dissimilarity measuring the gender employment gap has remained between 55 and 60 since 1950 [8]. The gender gap in work-related eye injuries, however, has been reported as even more skewed, at 98.8% for men and just 1.2% for women [20]. Simply put, industrial workers are disproportionately male, and even accounting for this imbalance, men are more likely to sustain ocular injuries in these fields. Victims of industrial eye accidents who were not wearing eye protection – a condition usually admitted by anywhere from 39.6% to 84.6% of the affected [20] – cite beliefs that eye protection is unnecessary, interferes with work performance, or is uncomfortable [3]. Military studies, dealing with a similar culture of masculinity, make a substantially more blunt prognosis, describing the infantryman, comparable to "another industrial worker needing eye protection," as – "young, emmetropic, unsophisticated, skeptical, denial-practicing, and body-image-conscious" [15] – i.e. sensitive to the age-old stigma that nerds, not real men, wear glasses. Not all of these concerns are unfounded, however, as a study of young, healthy volunteer subjects showed that wear of ANSI Z87.1- compliant eyewear diminished postural stability especially on an uneven standing surface [33]. Ongoing efforts to design more ergonomic and attractive protective equipment continue and are discussed below.

In theory, these stigmas, aversions, and economic obstacles could be addressed at the workplace level through comprehensive provision of protective eyewear, training in its use, and enforcement of its use. Unfortunately, even in the United Kingdom, where national legislation mandates the implementation of all three such stages, a workers' survey reported just 40% awareness/availability at the provision stage, and 20% conductance at the training stage [30].

Industrial Injuries: Standards and Enforcement

In the United States, the Occupational Safety and Health Administration (OSHA) is responsible for enforcing eye protection standards and regulation. Protective eyewear standards first began to be codified in the US in 1922, when the National Bureau of Standards, in consultation with the War and Navy Departments, issued the Z2 standard for head and eye protection, primarily addressing exposure to dust and fumes. Until 1961, the Z2 was revised on average once every decade, incorporating respiratory standards in 1938, and the advent of plastic materials in 1948 [1]. At that time, eye protection was transferred to its own standard, the Z87, which continues to be adjusted to this day, most recently in 2010 and 2015, and covers protective spectacles, goggles, welding helmets, faceshields, and anything else related to eye protection. A significant change in the 2010 edition was the introduction of standards for extent of eye coverage as well as introduction of more widely used test head models [1].

While the 2015 standard is still being adopted in some industries, the 2010 standard is codified in US safety regulations, and as of 2016, OSHA orders that employers provide personal protective eyewear to employees exposed to "flying particles, molten metal, liquid chemicals, acids or caustic liquids, chemical gases or vapors, or potentially injurious radiation." [32]. In turn, the American National Standards Institute (ANSI) and the International Safety Equipment Association (ISEA) are responsible for developing the exact standards for individual eyewear units, based on the recommendations of a panel of representatives from the optical, industrial, manufacturing, and military fields [1]. To comply with the ANSI/ISEA standards, all protective eyewear must meet standards in optical (addressing requirements such as minimal transmission and maximum astigmatism) and physical (addressing requirements such as coverage area, proper ventilation, and lens thickness) categories [1]. Based on exposed hazards, protective eyewear also must meet requirements in other categories such as radiation protection (including automatic darkening and filtering), or droplet/splash hazards (including occlusion to liquid and fine dust particles) [32].

As part of its pre-European Union move to establish an internal continental market, the European Commission established uniform health and safety requirements for all personal protective equipment, including protective eyewear, in December of 1989, in the form of a directive of ambiguous binding status [7]. The European Commission continues to maintain these standards, attempting to regulate both economic and safety questions. In general, the safety standards outlined are quite similar to the ANSI/ISEA standards, with the addition of manufacturing inspection standards. Under recent European Parliament action, the European Commission directive will be repealed in 2018 and replaced by a new set of regulations, ostensibly designed to increase conformity in manufacturing [26].

The status of standards and enforcement is less clear in the rest of the world. The efficacy such programs is difficult to determine even in India and China, both of which have been at the forefront of the developing world in terms of standard creation and enforcement. India's standards for industrial eye hazards and eyewear selection appear to have gone unchanged since 1977 although they were reaffirmed in 2002. They cover the same danger categories and the US and EU standards, but with unclear strictness and/or testing procedures [10]. China has conducted its own extensive government research on laser hazards to eye and other organ systems, although implementation seems to have focused on regulating hazard sources rather than human hazard protection [36].

The occupational health and vision screening aspects of industrial ophthalmology are beyond the scope of this chapter, and the reader is directed to an excellent overview of this topic by Blais [5].

Professional Sports Injuries

To sports fans and the observant public at large, eye injuries in professional sports occupy a category of unacceptability that transcends even unsettling "normal" trauma such as cuts and contusions. While fans consider Derek Jeter bloodying his chin launching himself into the seats at nearly 20 mph to catch a foul ball inspiring, they are appalled and nauseated when Juan Encarnación takes a foul ball to the orbit.

Unfortunately, the viewing public has witnessed many sports-related tragic eye injury incidents over the last several decades. Some of these injuries have ended careers, and others have led to campaigns for additional safety equipment. Some of the most prominent examples, culled from various sports, follow:

August 18, 1967, baseball: Boston Red Sox outfielder Tony Conigliaro was struck in the left periorbital area by a pitch from Jack Hamilton of the California Angels. Wearing an old-style batting helmet lacking an ear flap, Conigliaro had acute vision loss in the left eye and subsequently was diagnosed with traumatic macular hole. This injury resulted in poor depth perception and effectively ended his career. By 1983, Major League Baseball (MLB) mandated the use of a batting helmet with an ear flap facing the pitcher.

December 13, 2002, softball squash: Canada's Jonathon Power was hit accidentally in the left eye by an errant racquet move from his opponent David Palmer during their semifinal at the world championships [37]. Due to bleeding and periocular edema that did not allow him to open the eye, Power, the second-ranked player in the world, was forced to withdraw. Other players have suffered more serious and vision-threatening consequences such as retinal tear or detachment from such injuries, and Power was fortunate to escape with superficial injury alone [6]. Power was not wearing any eye protection during the match; competitors at the international senior level continue to be permitted to, and favor, wearing no eye protection, although polycarbonate goggles are required at the youth and collegiate levels internationally, and at the senior level in the United States.

March 5, 2013, ice hockey: New York Rangers' defenseman Marc Staal, wearing a helmet (mandatory since 1979) but not a visor, had a deflected slap shot impact his right orbital area. The resulting orbital fracture and traumatic retinal tear ended his season. Following his injury, Staal actively campaigned for a mandatory visor requirement in the National Hockey League (NHL), which was adopted beginning with the following (2013–2014) season, although players active before that season retain the right to go without a visor if they so choose. Even before the regulation took effect, visor use increased from 32% in the 2002–2003 season to 73% by the 2012–2013 season, and players who do not wear a visor are at over fourfold increased risk of incurring an eye or orbital injury [23]. There is some evidence that more skilled players have a higher rate of visor use [24], and as youth players look to these players as role models, they will hopefully see visor use in a positive light.

Military Eye Protection

The modern military poses a very interesting case study for the timely development, adoption, and future of eye protection devices. The need for credible eye protection in military settings is statistically clear and intuitive – according to an observational study of Israeli Defense Force records, eye injuries account for approximately 8–13% of battle-related injuries, despite the eye's comprising about 0.1% of body surface area [9]. This rate marks only the latest uptick in a worrisome trend, following such markers as estimated 0.5%, 2.0%, and 9.0% ocular injury shares during the US Civil War, both World Wars, and the Vietnam War respectively [15].

Furthermore, in terms of severity, 62.5% of the eye injuries in the Israeli study involved ballistic fragmentation and globe penetration, and 66% of such injuries (41.25% of all eye injuries) resulted in the victim being declared no longer fit for combat duty [9]. These figures reveal a minimal reduction in ultimate disability over the past 45 years of combat operations around the world, as 50% of American soldiers who suffered a penetrating eye injury in Vietnam ultimately lost the affected eye, even when receiving immediate and quality care [15].

As in industrial settings, though not quite as pronounced, increased use of eye protection appears to result in a significant decrease in ocular injury occurrence.

An American military study of eye injuries among 3276 casualties for whom eye protection status was known, during Operation Iraqi Freedom and Operation Enduring Freedom from 2004 to 2006, reported that 17% (451/2671) of those wearing eye protection vs. 26% (155/605) of those not wearing eye protection had an ocular injury ($p < 0.01$) [29]. An earlier study of ocular injuries during Operations Desert Shield and Desert Storm found that 40% of corneoscleral lacerations were caused by fragments <10 mm in size, and the authors postulated that the majority of these objects would have been stopped by polycarbonate eye protection [21] Retrospective analysis of ocular injuries in the Vietnam War estimated a 39% reduction in morbidity had even basic 2 mm polycarbonate lenses been available at the time [14].

Despite the clear demonstration of efficacy, these statistics have not necessarily bolstered rates of eye protection adoption within the armed forces. Concerns over scratches from sand or other particulate matter, restrictions of the field of vision due to poor design, basic complaints of being too hot or too bulky, the inaccurate perception of being in relative safety, or even fear of social stigma over wearing glasses of any form, can prompt servicemen to remove their eyewear [15]. The American service member appears particularly convinced of the negative potential on visual function from eye protection, and US military history is riddled with attempts at protective eyewear that have run into one or more of these objections.

The need for and development of eye protection for warfare has long focused on two major sources of risk, divided into: (1) hazards derived from the operational environment that impede vision, and (2) ballistic injuries sustained during simulated or real combat scenarios. On one hand, the first category encompasses strictly environmental perils like fine particular matter such as dirt and sand that scratch eye and eyewear alike, potentially resulting in incapacitation from corneal abrasions or the risk-inducing removal of eyewear, respectively [15]. It also includes man-made hazards not involving immediate combat, such as laser aids and flashes from high-powered (i.e. nuclear) weaponry [35]. The second is comprised of injuries resulting from threats roughly analogous to the high-velocity particle motion criterion previously discussed for sports and heavy industry, the difference being that in this case, the high-velocity particles in question are weaponized projectiles – bullets and fragments produced by explosions.

Additionally, although injuries from chemical warfare fail to fit neatly into either category, they have a demonstrated ability to cause debilitating ocular injuries. Sulfur mustard (bis(2-chloroethyl) sulfide), also known as mustard gas, one of the earliest and most notorious of chemical warfare agents, can irritate the eye at concentrations as low as 100 ppm, substantially lower than the concentration at which exposed skin reacts to the gas [35]. Exposure to mustard gas can cause corneal stromal inflammation and later permanent scarring, and this particular injury was not uncommon during gas warfare in the trenches of World War I, when the rarely-used American eye protection was a heavy metal face mask with open slits for eyes [15].

The pressing need for effective military eye protection was further acknowledged when advances in protection of other body areas both reduced injury risk to those areas and improved survival from previously fatal trauma. Most prominently, advances in body armor, in particular heavy-plate ceramic armor like the US Army's Improved Outer Tactical Vest (IOTV) that provides an unprecedented level of protection for vital organs, are contributing to increased survival rates even in situations such as IED detonations. Data from Operation Iraqi Freedom echo findings from the IDF [9], with ocular injury being the second most common bodily injury after amputation (although traumatic brain injury and post-traumatic stress disorder were, overall, more frequent than eye trauma) [34]. Even prototypes of the futuristic Tactical Assault Light Operator Suit (TALOS) for special operations – hyped with Iron Man comparisons and featuring self-healing and instantaneously hardening liquid body armor – have only marginal improvements to safety in the ocular area [16].

The future development of military eye protection will be calibrated to provide even more of a defense against the two previously-listed major threats – ballistic fragmentation and operationally challenging terrain and variable weather conditions of wartime environments – plus growing concerns over laser damage.

Efforts to increase ballistic fragmentation resistance are focused on modifying the polycarbonate lenses and frames that have become the staple components of impact-resistant eyewear. Researchers at the US Army Natick Soldier Research, Development and Engineering Center (NSRDEC) have worked to incorporate proprietary blends of nylon materials into spectacle lenses; such materials have heretofore been used in spectacle frames but not lenses. Preliminary results indicate a 15–20% improvement in impact resistance as well as overall reduction in the weight of the eyewear [4].

Laser-resistant eyewear would be taking on a critical timeline even if increased battlefield usage of aids such as laser-based range finders and target designators were the sole impetus. The prospect of the long-anticipated transition of laser weaponry from science fiction into real-life warfare has only accelerated the need, as evidenced by the 30 kW test AN/SEQ-3 laser weapon system installed on the USS *Ponce*, and Lockheed Martin's revealed plans to manufacture 60 kW lasers for inclusion in directed-energy weapons on the new F-35 fighter jet [18].

Setting the laser weapons of the future aside for the moment, even the standard laser aiming systems of current artillery rangefinders can cause flash blindness/dazzle, corneal edema, or severe retinal burns and choroidal hemorrhages, due to the high degree of focusing by the eye that can decrease the effective diameter of a laser spot to 10–20 μm and magnify the energy density by a factor of 10^5 [11]. Currently, in the military and industry alike, laser protective eyewear uses either an implanted absorptive dye, effective across only a restrictive wavelength range, or an optical filter layer, similarly constrained in range. Military research now centers on trying to eliminate this reliance on different tints or filters for different wavelengths of light, leading optimally to an adaptive, single-lens system. No operational system exists currently.

To address one perennial environmental hazard, variable lighting conditions, fast-tint protective eyewear (FTPE), has been proposed as the future eye protection of the Navy SEALS. FTPE takes ordinary transitional lenses – such as the common prescription eyeglasses that gradually darken to act as sunglasses when exposed to ultraviolet energy – and expands the tinting options while cutting the transition time by using LCD technology. In less than half a second, an electric impulse, applied manually or automatically, causes the constituent liquid crystal solution to adopt one of three hues or a clear output in accordance with light in the surroundings. In contrast, transitional lenses can take several minutes to darken with UV exposure and return to clarity when UV light is withdrawn. FTPE units will be produced to the same ballistics standards as existing combat goggles, but with an appearance and weight similar to sports sunglasses (Office of Naval Research, unpublished information). Other work at NSRDEC seeks to address the most common complaints from soldiers about protective eyewear – scratches from sand and greatly reduced vision in fog – by developing new goggle coatings.

Civilian Accidental Trauma

Looking outside of industry for similar injuries in a civilian setting, three categories stand out – pyrotechnics-related, arms-related, and amateur sports-related – all sharing the high-velocity, high-momentum, and/or high-temperature characteristics of the aforementioned accident-prone industrial contexts.

According to retroactive analyses of two eye injury registries (Eye Injury Registry of Alabama and the Hungarian Eye Injury Registry), approximately 4.4% of reported eye injuries between January, 1980 and December, 1997 were fireworks-related, with no use of eye protection in any reported incident, injuries to both perpetrators and bystanders, and an especially high rate of injury to young males [13]. In both children and adults, burns to the hand are the most common injury from fireworks; however, children may be at even higher risk of eye injuries than adults when handling fireworks, as a study during Diwali in New Delhi reported 65 cases of pediatric fireworks-related injuries in which 21 (32%) involved the face and 7 (11%) involved the eyes [2]. Data from the US Centers for Disease Control and Prevention (CDC) corroborate these findings, with injuries to the eyes as the second-most-commonly reported injury in US fireworks-related scenarios, trailing only hand and finger injuries [31]. While burns from fireworks are the most-common reported injury on an overall basis (54.3% of all cases, again according to the CDC), eye injuries are unique in featuring a high rate of non-burn injuries including, but not limited to, contusions and lacerations (84.6%). In a 6-year survey of fireworks-related eye injuries in northern China, eyelid laceration and orbital fracture were the most common injuries seen; multiple ocular injuries were not uncommon, and corneoscleral laceration repair was required in 35 of 99 patients as was vitrectomy in 33 [12]. Final visual outcome was counting fingers or worse in 42.9% of all 105 injured eyes [12]. While eye protection status was not reported systematically, its use rarely occurs or is encouraged by amateur fireworks users.

While firearms are a concern for military eye injuries, civilians are more likely to incur eye injuries from pressure-driven weapons such as air, BB, and paintball guns – all of which deserve particular emphasis for their injury rates among children.

A 1994 study using eye injury registry data reported a median age of 13 in air gun eye accidents, with an adult present in only 14/130 (11%) of cases where a child was injured [28]. A 2012 study from a tertiary care hospital reported 3161 emergency room visits for children suffering eye injuries in nonpowder gun-related injuries, and only 1 in 71 patients was wearing eye protection at the time of injury [17]. The same authors reported a trend of decreasing paintball-related injuries but increasing air gun-related injuries [17]. In the United States, the fear of liability and lawsuits has led commercial paintball and air gun facility operators to require eye protection use, but these rules do not apply to individuals when they are on their own property or elsewhere. Though air guns have been marketed as a safer alternative to BB guns due to their use of plastic pellets rather than metal ones, the occurrence of ocular penetration injuries, oftentimes resulting in post-surgery visual acuity or 20/200 is worse, is greater for air guns [28].

Civilian recreation and sporting activities deserve a note in part for their differences from the "industrial" level of professional sports in terms of safety attitudes and measures. For instance, looking back at the three specific examples of famous professional sports injuries, youth levels of each enforce safety measures to reduce the same exact risks: Little League Baseball required two-earflap batting helmets beginning in 1958, youth squash players (through U19) are required to wear polycarbonate goggles at the international level, and all non-adult participants in USA Hockey-sanctioned events must wear facemasks (even more encompassing than visors). However, in some sports, such as lacrosse, cultural attitudes on gender continue to affect eye protection rules, with eyewear required for women's competitions, but merely recommended for men's. Still, despite higher safety standards at youth levels, many of which have been in place for decades, about one-third of the >100,000 annual civilian sports-related injuries and their associated $175 million price tag are pediatric [25]. Improper fit of protective wear in children remains a challenge, and the cost of replacing protective gear as a child grows can be a substantial barrier to its proper acquisition and use.

Conclusions

Eye protection in hazardous environments remains challenging. Cultural and practical barriers impede the widespread use of eye protection in heavy industry despite regulations that have been issued over the years. Failure to train workers in the use of protective equipment and even the lack of the equipment itself leads to preventable injuries that can cost workers their livelihood. Similarly, high-profile accidents have ended the careers of professional athletes, but using eye protection at the elite levels of competition remains options in many sports. Taking advantage of its hierarchical culture, the military has had some success in reducing eye injuries by mandating use of eye protection in combat and training environments. Finally, children remain the disproportionate victims of civilian ballistic eye injuries, and further efforts are needed to identify the best methods to protect them from these largely avoidable insults.

Compliance with Ethical Requirements Arjuna M. Subramanian and Prem S. Subramanian declare that they have no conflict of interest. No human or animal studies were carried out by the authors for this chapter.

References

1. American National Standard for Occupational and Educational Personal Eye and Face Protection Devices. American National Standard for occupational and educational personal eye and face protection devices. Arlington: International Safety Equipment Association; 2010.
2. Bagri N, Saha A, Chandelia S, Dubey NK, Bhatt A, Rai A, Bhattacharya S, Makhija LK. Fireworks injuries in children: a prospective study during the festival of lights. Emerg Med Australas. 2013;25:452–6. doi:10.1111/1742-6723.12114.
3. Banerjee A. Effectiveness of eye protection in the metal working industry. BMJ: Br Med J. 1990;301:645–6.
4. Benson, J. Natick takes protective eyewear into the future | [WWW Document]. armytech-nology.armylive.dodlive.mil. 2014. URL http://armytechnology.armylive.dodlive.mil/index.php/2014/05/01/9/. Accessed 1.22.17.
5. Blais BR. Basic principles of industrial ophthalmology. Ophthalmol Clin N Am. 1999;12:303–32. doi:10.1016/S0896-1549(05)70110-3.
6. Carlin W. Will Carlin's experience with being hit | Squash Magazine [WWW Document]. 2014. squashmagazine.ussquash.com. URL http://squashmagazine.ussquash.com/2014/02/will-carlins-experience-with-being-hit/. Accessed 1.2.17.
7. Council Directive of 21 December 1989 on the approximation of the laws of the Member States relating to personal protective equipment (89/686/EEC). Off J Eur Commun. 1989.
8. England P. The gender revolution. Gend Soc. 2010;24:149–66. doi:10.1177/0891243210361475.
9. Gendler S, Nadler R, Erlich T, Fogel O, Shushan G, Glassberg E. Eye injury in the Israeli defense force: an ounce of prevention is worth a pound of cure. Injury. 2015;46:1241–5.
10. Guide for selection of industrial safety equipment for eye, face, and ear protection. New Delhi: Indian Standards Institution; 1977.
11. Harris MD, Lincoln AE, Amoroso PJ, Stuck B, Sliney D. Laser eye injuries in military occupations. Aviat Space Environ Med. 2003;74:947–52.
12. Kong Y, Tang X, Kong B, Jiang H, Chen Y. Six-year clinical study of firework-related eye injuries in North China. Postgrad Med J. 2015;91:26–9. doi:10.1136/postgradmedj-2014-132837.
13. Kuhn FC, Morris RC, Witherspoon DC, Mann L, Mester V, Módis L, Berta A, Bearden W. Serious fireworks-related eye injuries. Ophthalmic Epidemiol. 2000;7:139–48. doi:10.1076/0928-6586(200006)721-ZFT139.
14. La Piana FG, Hornblass A. Military ophthalmology in the Vietnam war. Doc Ophthalmol. 1997;93:29–48. doi:10.1007/BF02569045.
15. La Piana FG, Ward TP. The development of eye armor for the American infantryman. Ophthalmol Clin N Am. 1999;12:421–34. doi:10.1016/S0896-1549(05)70118-8.
16. Lanaria V. U.S. military to deliver its first bulletproof, weaponized iron man suit in 2018 [WWW Document]. 2016. URL http://www.techtimes.com/articles/92478/20151007/u-s-military-to-deliver-its-first-bulletproof-weaponized-iron-man-suit-in-2018.htm. Accessed 1.23.17.
17. Lee R, Fredrick D. Pediatric eye injuries due to nonpowder guns in the United States, 2002–2012. J AAPOS. 2015;19:163–168.e1. doi:10.1016/j.jaapos.2015.01.010.
18. Leopold G. How lasers could make the F-35 more effective [WWW Document]. defensesystems.com. 2015. URL https://defensesystems.com/articles/2016/09/01/f35-lasers-marines-joint-strike-fighter.aspx. Accessed 1.23.17.

19. Lombardi DA, Pannala R, Sorock GS, Wellman H, Courtney TK, Verma S, Smith GS. Welding related occupational eye injuries: a narrative analysis. Inj Prev. 2005;11:174–9. doi:10.1136/ip.2004.007088.
20. MacEwen CJ. Eye injuries: a prospective survey of 5671 cases. Br J Ophthalmol. 1989;73:888–94.
21. Mader TH, Aragones JV, Chandler AC, Hazlehurst JA, Heier J, Kingham JD, Stein E. Ocular and ocular adnexal injuries treated by United States military ophthalmologists during operations desert shield and desert storm. Ophthalmology. 1993;100:1462–7. doi:10.1016/S0161-6420(93)31455-7.
22. May DR, Kuhn FC, Morris RE, Witherspoon CD, Danis RP, Matthews GP, Mann L. The epidemiology of serious eye injuries from the United States eye injury registry. Graefes Arch Clin Exp Ophthalmol. 2000;238:153–7.
23. Micieli JA, Zurakowski D, Ahmed IIK. Impact of visors on eye and orbital injuries in the National Hockey League. Can J Ophthalmol. 2014;49:243–8. doi:10.1016/j.jcjo.2014.03.008.
24. Micieli R, Micieli JA. Visor use among National Hockey League players and its relationship to on-ice performance. Inj Prev. 2016;22:392–5. doi:10.1136/injuryprev-2015-041900.
25. Napier SM, Baker RS, Sanford DG, Easterbrook M. Eye injuries in athletics and recreation. Surv Ophthalmol. 1996;41:229–44.
26. Regulation (EU) 2016/425 of the European Parliament and of the Council. Regulation (EU) 2016/425 of the European Parliament and of the Council. Off J Eur Union. 2016.
27. Saari KM, Parvi V. Occupational eye injuries in Finland. Acta Ophthalmol. 1984;62:17–28. doi:10.1111/j.1755-3768.1984.tb06779.x.
28. Schein OD, Enger C, Tielsch JM. The context and consequences of ocular injuries from air guns. Am J Ophthalmol. 1994;117:501–6.
29. Thomas R, McManus JG, Johnson A, Mayer P, Wade C, Holcomb JB. Ocular injury reduction from ocular protection use in current combat operations. J Trauma. 2009;66:S99–S103. doi:10.1097/ta.0b013e31819d8695.
30. Thompson GJ, Mollan SP. Occupational eye injuries: a continuing problem. Occup Med (Lond). 2009;59:123–5. doi:10.1093/occmed/kqn168.
31. Tu Y, Granados DV. Fireworks annual report. United States Government, Washington, DC; 2014.
32. Updating OSHA Standards Based on National Consensus Standards; Eye and Face Protection. Final rule. Updating OSHA standards based on National Consensus standards; eye and face protection. Final rule. Fed Regist. 2016;81:16085–93.
33. Wade L, Weimar W, Davis J. Effect of personal protective eyewear on postural stability. Ergonomics. 2004;47:1614–23. doi:10.1080/00140130410001724246.
34. Weichel ED, Colyer MH. Combat ocular trauma and systemic injury. Curr Opin Ophthalmol. 2008;19:519–25. doi:10.1097/ICU.0b013e3283140e98.
35. Wong TY, Seet MB, Ang CL. Eye injuries in twentieth century warfare: a historical perspective. Surv Ophthalmol. 1997;41:433–59.
36. Yigao J. People's Republic of China laser radiation safety standard. Dayton, United States Government, Washington DC; 1989.
37. Zug J. Thirty years on: the history of eye protection in the U.S. l Squash Magazine [WWW Document]. squashmagazine.ussquash.com. 2014. URL http://squashmagazine.ussquash.com/2014/02/thirty-years-on-the-history-of-eye-protection-in-the-u-s-by-james-zug/. Accessed 1.2.17.

Index

© Springer International Publishing AG 2017

P.S. Subramanian (ed.), *Ophthalmology in Extreme Environments*,
Essentials in Ophthalmology, DOI 10.1007/978-3-319-57600-8